Thank You for All of Your Help and Support
Compliments of
Breast Cancer Help, Inc.
Long Island Cancer Help and Wellness Center

MAP OF DESTINY

Pinpointing a Cancer Epidemic on the Kitchen Table

Joan Swirsky

Tempest Books
Forest Hills, New York

Notice

Map of Destiny is based on the professional background, personal experiences, and research of the author, who has tried to portray as accurately as possible the story of the efforts of Lorraine Pace and her colleagues to map the incidence of breast cancer in West Islip, New York, as well as to detail the history of the breast cancer advocacy movement that flourished on Long Island during the 1990s. The initial publication of *Map of Destiny* involves a limited number of soft cover copies and CD-ROMs.   If any reader detects any *factual* inaccuracies, please contact the author immediately at www.mapofdestiny.com to be sure that future versions include the appropriate changes.

This book is dedicated to all the heroic breast cancer patients on Long Island whose relentless and passionate activism has brought the entire world closer to understanding – and potentially curing – the merciless scourge of breast cancer.

And to my husband, Steve, for his endless encouragement, support and love.

CONTENTS

ACKNOWLEDGMENTS

In loving memory of my publisher, Howard Kane, who died suddenly on the eve of this book's publication but whose tireless help, eternal optimism, sage advice and intense interest helped immeasurably in bringing Map of Destiny from computer page to publication.

To Marcia Kane Hittner, who has continued her father's work, bringing her own unique personal qualities and business talents to this project.

To Jerome Pittman for his unflagging computer work and beautiful cover art.

To Rita Samols, my brilliant and generous editor.

INTRODUCTION

Cancer. Cancer. Cancer.

On Long Island, where I live, this word rolls off the tongue as commonly as McDonald's, the Dow and the latest Washington high jinks. On this relatively small strip of land, containing fewer than three million people, cancer is a fact of life for far too many.

It is certainly not a subject that people seek out. I didn't. Cancer found me. Not as a patient but as a journalist who was assigned a single article in 1985 and became so infuriated by what I learned that simple, energizing rage compelled me to dig deeper.

At that time, a small article in *Newsday*, Long Island's only daily newspaper, reported on breast cancer incidence in Long Island's two counties. It stated that in Nassau County, the rate was 112.6 cases per 100,000 women per year, or 18.9 percent above the state average and 30 percent higher than the national average; in Suffolk County the rate was 103.6 cases per 100,000, or 9.4 percent above the state average of 89.5 per 100,000.

In short, the incidence of breast cancer in both Nassau and Suffolk counties was significantly higher than it was throughout the state, in neighboring Queens, or in nearby Westchester County, which has a demographic profile strikingly similar to that of Long Island.

Worse, state health officials had known these statistics for 10 years and had done nothing to implement a study. As far back as 1979, Dr. Andre Varma, a professor of community and preventive medicine at the State University of New York Stony Brook, was alarmed by the breast cancer incidence and, in 1982, proposed a study. But it took another two years – to write a grant, apply for funding, coordinate various agencies, and deal with the clashing egos of the participants – before the study got off the ground.

Finally, in early 1985, a collaborative study by the New York State Department of Health, the State University of New York at Stony Brook, and the health departments of Nassau and Suffolk counties was begun. So poorly funded was the study, however, that everyone involved – epidemiologists, physicians, surveyors, and pathologists – was volunteering his or her services. In fact, the participants were picking up the bill!

My publisher at the time, Jane Gitlin, had just founded a monthly newspaper, *The Women's Record*, with the goal of addressing the educational, business, and medical concerns of women. Although the paper had a relatively small circulation, its mailing list included all of Long Island's shakers and movers: politicians, educators, physicians, and business people. My assignment was to find out what the breast cancer problem was all about.

"Simple," I thought. With my nursing background, I anticipated that my search for and understanding of clinical information would be uncomplicated, and that by contacting the "experts" in medicine and epidemiology, the mystery of Long Island's high incidence of breast cancer would be clarified.

But that isn't what happened. From the outset, it was clear that the people from the county and state health departments who I believed were in a position to give me answers either could not or did not want to. And the doctors I spoke with seemed mystified by the great number of women they were seeing with breast cancer, some shrugging in helplessness as they tried to explain the phenomenon, others guessing – off the record – that it might be "something" in the environment.

In short, I was asking a lot of questions but getting no closer to understanding why so many women in our region were getting this dread disease. Then I decided to visit the Nassau County Board of Health to question not only the high incidence of breast cancer but also why there seemed to be so many clusters of the disease in certain neighborhoods.

"Do you keep track of every woman who gets breast cancer, and of the clusters?" I asked one of the higher-ups there. "And where do these statistics go?"

He told me yes, the department did keep track, and no, there were no clusters. Then he showed me a map. "Look here," he said. "Every pin you see on this map denotes a case of cancer in our county."

That was when I knew that the solitary article I had been assigned to write would be insufficient to cover what to me appeared to be at best a very serious unsolved mystery and at worst a cover-up. The map was situated so high up on the wall and blanketed with so many tiny multicolored pins that even someone using binoculars couldn't have made sense of it. And the "there are no clusters" statement flew in the face of the many neighborhoods I had visited in which three, five, even nine women on one block had breast cancer.

Moreover, I learned that the state's cancer registry was hopelessly outdated, with literally years of files sitting in cardboard boxes waiting to be recorded by secretaries who would ultimately type the information into a database. That's right: even in the mid-1980s the system was not computerized!

The one article I was assigned turned into a series of eight articles covering the clinical, emotional, environmental, and political aspects of breast cancer. Because I was writing for a small, independent newspaper led by a publisher who spurred my efforts on, I was able to engage in a form of "advocacy" journalism, not only reporting "the facts" but also challenging the design of the New York State study, the apathy of politicians, the neglect of environmental issues, and the patronizing medical policies that made women the very last people to participate in their own health-care decisions.

The eight articles grew into 200 articles over a period of 15 years, not only for *The Women's Record* but also for *Merrick Life*, *Networking*, other regional newspapers, and the Long Island section of *The New York Times*.

Introduction

Some people began to take notice. The late state Senator Michael J. Tully Jr., beginning in 1984, was the first politician to advocate for – and get enacted – some of the most cutting-edge breast cancer legislation in the nation, including a law mandating that doctors tell women *all* their treatment options when they are diagnosed with the disease.

My newspaper took action as well. After the initial analysis of the Stony Brook study was released in 1986, reporting only on "known" risk factors for breast cancer (i.e., age, family history, ethnic background, age at first childbirth, etc.), there seemed to be a thundering silence about the study for months and months on end.

Disgusted that a follow-up analysis of the study had not been released in two years, *The Women's Record* spearheaded a write-in campaign in June of 1988 that resulted in 3,000 letters being delivered to the chairman of the state Senate Standing Committee on Health, Tarky Lombardi, in Albany.

A couple of weeks later – not coincidentally, we believed – a press conference was held on Long Island at which an analysis was finally presented by Dr. Philip Nasca, the director of the state health department's Bureau of Epidemiology. He cited "30 years of studies indicating there is no relationship between breast cancer and environmental factors" and stated that the Long Island study had revealed no new information about the disease. It did not escape the attention of those present that the study had failed to ask women about two important variables: their sources of drinking water and their proximity to the many toxic dumpsites and landfills that dotted Long Island.

Dr. Nasca's pronouncements were greeted with skepticism and anger by people who were aware that a great number of Long Island's monitoring wells – which, unlike pumping wells, collect water samples to test for the presence of physical, chemical, or biological contaminants – had been closed or restricted because of systemic organic chemical or nitrate contamination; that the Old Bethpage landfill was considered the number one toxic dumpsite in New York state by the Environmental Protection Agency; that the fumes from other landfills were suspected of making schoolchildren sick; that one community's groundwater was found to have concentrations of carcinogenic chemicals 2,400 times higher than state Health Department guidelines; and that a 1985 issue of *Connoisseur Magazine* had ranked Long Island's water as among the worst in the nation.

Dr. Nasca's words also fueled my own resolve to keep demanding, in print, that the study – or *some* study – include environmental data. The investigators closed the press conference by promising to release additional data in 1990.

In the interim, Senator Tully became the chairman of the state health committee and continued to fight for and enact breast cancer legislation that included adding insurance coverage for diagnostic mammography, lowering the age of insurance coverage for mammography from 49 to 40, instituting a statewide breast cancer advisory board, and appropriating $1 million for a statewide breast cancer detection and education program.

In addition, the Nassau County Executive, Thomas J. Gulotta, mandated that every woman in the county be given a free mammogram, a program that still exists and is the only one of its kind in the nation. And *The Women's Record* initiated another write-in campaign, which yielded 12,000 signatures, to urge New York State legislators to code by census tract all cases of breast cancer on Long Island for the previous five years, data that could reveal information on approximately 8,000 cases instead of the 1,400 that the Stony Brook study had looked at.

The response was immediate: Senator Tully and State Assemblyman Tom DiNapoli introduced legislation calling for geocoding of breast cancer cases by census tract not simply for the previous five years but for the previous 10 years – or 14,000 cases! This would allow investigators to break down the addresses in each census area (by county, postal route, etc.) in order to compare their demographics more precisely.

On October 22, 1990, after the Long Island study had been redesigned twice – to include more questions about the environment and a look at breast cancer cases over the previous 10 years – another press conference was held at Stony Brook.

This time, Dr. Nasca told the audience that questions about the environment had been included in the study but, after looking at the relationship of the subjects' disease to contaminated wells and hazardous waste sites, they had ruled out environmental factors. In fact, every one of the several breast cancer patients I interviewed who had participated in the study by answering the questionnaire reported they had *never* been asked about their sources of drinking water or their proximity to toxic dumpsites!

Dr. Nasca's conclusion also enraged Faith Laursen, a breast cancer survivor and the owner of *Merrick Life* and three other South Shore newspapers. And it angered her daughter, Linda Toscano, *Merrick Life's* publisher, who had reported widely on the breast cancer problem and had published a lengthy questionnaire in the newspaper that revealed "hot spots" of the disease in both residential areas and workplaces.

More infuriating to the breast cancer survivors and advocates who attended the press conference was Dr. Nasca's conclusion. "Based on this investigation, no additional studies by the New York State Department of Health are warranted," he said, and took his leave.

Unwittingly, he had let the horse of public outrage out of the barn, and it would not be long before grassroots groups would rise up to lobby for a truly comprehensive study of breast cancer vis-à-vis the environment on Long Island.

Just when I thought that the grassroots advocates had thought of and were fighting for everything that was crucial to finding a cause and cure for breast cancer – everything from public awareness about the importance of early detection to raising funds for research into the genetic and biological roots of the disease to lobbying for new legislation – I met Lorraine Pace.

Introduction

From the moment I spoke to Lorraine and saw her "in action," I knew that she had come upon a better mousetrap in breast cancer advocacy. I felt that Lorraine's story was so important that I called my editor at the *Times*, Stewart Kampel, and arranged to meet him in New York City to explain the importance of Lorraine's story.

He listened. He nodded. He suggested that I include in the article a few other people who had "taken matters into their own hands," and he gave me the okay to go ahead.

On July 5, 1992, my 4,000-word article was published and, as Lorraine would say, "The rest is history." The next day she received calls from CNN, ABC-TV, and *USA Today*. In the weeks and months and years that followed, she was contacted by just about every other news organization in the country, featured in hundreds of articles and made TV and radio appearances too numerous to list.

Since that time, she has shared her "better mousetrap" idea with thousands upon thousands of people, all of whom feel – many for the first time in their lives – that they can finally take some semblance of control and embark on the right road to solving the mystery of the cancer surrounding them in their neighborhoods.

But this is Lorraine's story, the story of one woman going along, living her life, doing her thing, and then hit with the devastating lightning bolt of breast cancer, which changed her life forever. More than that, it is the story of a woman who refused to accept *anything* she was told about why she and so many of her Long Island neighbors had breast cancer, a woman who decided, in a very original way, to set about finding answers.

In so doing, she influenced individuals and organizations both inside and outside the United States to take matters into their own hands, inspired – and instructed – the grassroots groups on Long Island to follow her lead, and served as a major catalyst in convincing the most powerful science organization in the world – the National Cancer Institute – to undertake the most expensive and comprehensive study in its history to determine if there was a connection between breast cancer and the environment on Long Island.

Chapter One

"Life Is Good"

By the time most people reach the age of 50, they're already survivors. Even if their lives have been relatively untroubled, by that age just about everyone has been through some kind of mill: job searches and job losses, marriage and all of its attendant sacrifices and frustrations, the inevitable highs and lows of parenthood, and the deaths of loved ones. In other words, real life!

For Lorraine Pace, the thought of reaching the half-century mark and its well-deserved recognition of seasoning and maturity was a time of sober soul-searching as well as celebration. On the first day of June in 1991, she started to turn the page of the calendar that hung on the wall of her immaculate kitchen. It was a floral calendar, full of colorful bouquets of daisies, lilacs, dahlias – different flowers for each month and all in her favorite pastels.

She always hated to part with the previous month's picture, often removing it to mount on her bureau or frame for posterity. As she took one last look at May's dancing daffodils, she decided not to flip the page forward but instead to review the months that had elapsed since the beginning of the year.

Gazing at April's forsythias, Lorraine was transported back to her childhood in Brooklyn, where every street seemed ablaze with the flower's golden blossoms. She had once read that in 1940 the borough president, John Cashmore, had pronounced the forsythia Brooklyn's official flower, a symbol she thought fitting for the colorful, vibrant borough.

She smiled to herself as she remembered the bustling streets of her old neighborhood and the hordes of neighborhood children who swarmed about when the days were bright and a stickball game was the most important thing in the world. She recalled the sweltering summers and how she and her friends shrieked with delight when a swaggering teenager opened a fire hydrant and the water spewed into the air, splashing every passerby and even the mothers who sat fanning themselves on their stoops as they rocked their babies.

The apartments Lorraine lived in, though never very large, were always permeated with the warmth and personality of her Irish and English ancestors who lived nearby. Her father was the superintendent of many of the apartment houses, which spared them a monthly rent, but money was always tight. She and her brothers were expected to earn what they could, which Lorraine did by babysitting and selling the pot holders she made door to door.

As she stood in her kitchen, still absorbed by the forsythias, Lorraine felt very fortunate to be in exactly that place at exactly that moment. She found herself reflecting on her past, her parents, her life's accomplishments, the quite wonderful life she'd lived for the previous 30 years, and also on the impending occasion of, as she called it, "The Big Five O."

Spring had been a time of celebration. Lorraine and her husband, John, had attended the law school graduation of their daughter, Lisa Marie. John was a lawyer himself, and the fact that his daughter had followed in his footsteps was a source of great pride to him.

As if that weren't enough, their son Gregory had just graduated from Syracuse University and started work as a producer and senior program coordinator for YES TV in the Town of Islip's Youth Enrichment Services. And John Jr., a graduate of Fairfield University in Connecticut, was 29, living at home, and excelling professionally as the youthful head of Pace Real Estate Services.

All at once, Lorraine abandoned her reflections on things past and turned the page of her calendar forward to June and her thoughts to the historic occasion of her upcoming birthday. "Fifty," she thought to herself, "and here I am standing in my beautiful home and feeling great. My children are healthy and on their own. My husband is a good man, and I have a wonderful job. God, I'm lucky. Thank you, God. Life is good."

The sight of June's vase of radiant roses, however, turned her thoughts to the past once again. Lost in reverie, she remembered the day she moved to West Islip as a teenager and how astounded she was to look up at the heavens and see, not the smog and haze of the Brooklyn sky but the moon and stars in all of their sparkling splendor.

Warmed by the memory, she once again felt fortunate to have moved to a community with such an abundance of beautiful trees, pristine lakes, and clean air, a place where she and her friends swam in the summer and skated in the winter at Deer Lake, sat around campfires, attended dances for 10 cents, and threw last-minute come-as-you-are parties where the girls showed up in hair curlers and the boys in dungarees covered with car grease.

As if the advent of her upcoming birthday somehow required her to review her life, Lorraine thought back to her years at West Islip High School in the late 1950s, of being a gung-ho member of the Girls Leaders Club, planning social activities and even spearheading a fund-raising drive for the community's United Fund. She chuckled to herself remembering the back-flips and somersaults and splits she did in gymnastics, the hoops she scored in basketball, and the cold November day when her fingers almost froze playing the clarinet in the school's marching band.

Inevitably, her reminiscences led her to the day she was introduced to the man she would marry. A couple of months after finishing high school, she was convinced to attend an Italian-American Republican Club function by her friend Annie, who promised that two "eligible" young men would be there. Although she hesitated at first, afraid that her mother and father – Vivian and James Trim, both Democrats – would disapprove, she attended the affair and even allowed Annie to arrange a double date.

As was common in those times, however, a date could not take place before the Trims had met – and approved of – any potential suitor.

20

Lorraine didn't fall for John right away, but her mother took an immediate liking to him. It was eternally embarrassing to the young girl to see John sitting in her kitchen having pie and coffee with her mother while other boys picked her up for dates. She begged her mother to stop inviting the young lawyer to the house and, reluctantly, Vivian finally gave in to her daughter's demands.

But fate has a way of countering the embarrassment of daughters and the acquiescence of mothers. At the time, Lorraine was accustomed to driving to her job as a "candy girl" at Sears Roebuck and looking forward to her job as a stenographer at the Long Island State Park Commission. But one day, a car accident damaged her car so extensively that she had no way to get to work.

When John heard about the accident, he offered to drive Lorraine to work, and her mother hired him to represent Lorraine in a lawsuit arising from the accident. John won a judgment in Lorraine's favor, and he was so persuasive that he not only inspired Lorraine's parents to change their political affiliation from Democrat to Republican, he also convinced their daughter to marry him! In July of 1960, he and 19-year-old Lorraine announced their engagement.

In September, during a particularly devastating hurricane, Lorraine's father underwent major surgery – during a power outage! As the family waited anxiously for word that her father was okay, none of them were aware that the surgery was being performed using the hospital's generators or that her mother, while rushing up the stairs of the hospital, had suffered a major heart attack.

For the next two weeks, both of Lorraine's parents lay in guarded condition in the same critical-care ward. When they went home several weeks later, a semblance of normal life returned to the Trim household.

Relieved and once again feeling excited and carefree, Lorraine spent the next several months running from her job to wedding-gown fittings and the elaborate planning of her big day. The romance that almost wasn't was. With her mother having acted as a de facto matchmaker, John and Lorraine were married on July 22, 1961.

As Lorraine stood in her kitchen looking back on her life, she was flooded with thoughts of her mother. Vivian had married at 17 and always retained the blush of youth. Still in her teens, she had given birth to her first son, Ronald James. Although she came from a large family and was one of six siblings herself, Vivian's dream of filling her home with many children didn't materialize. As one year passed into another, she hoped and prayed for another baby, lighting candles in church in hopes of bringing about "the miracle," as she called her longed-for baby.

It wasn't for another nine and a half years that her prayers were answered; on June 30, 1941, little Lorraine made her debut. Less than two years later, Vivian gave birth again, to Lawrence.

Lorraine adored her baby brother, as did the whole family, but she always felt that it was her birth – not just as the only daughter but also after her mother had wanted for so many years to get pregnant – that gave her special status in the Trim household.

In later years, especially when Lorraine had her own three children, she would laugh when she remembered her mother saying that *each one* of her three children was her "favorite" – the oldest because he was the oldest, Lorraine because she was the only girl, the baby because he was the baby.

Lorraine thought back to her mother's energy and optimism, to the deep kindness and understanding she extended to just about everyone who crossed her path. She pictured her mother waving to the neighbors as she strode the streets of her Brooklyn neighborhood, her long blonde hair blowing in the breeze.

She could hear her mother's voice singing Irish folk songs as she pinned the wet laundry from the wicker basket onto the clotheslines that hung in the basement. Lorraine knew her mother regretted that her family's clothes didn't smell as "fresh-air clean" as her neighbor's clothes because their ground-floor apartment abutted a brick wall.

She imagined her mother bustling around their tiny kitchen seasoning her aromatic stews, stirring pots of steaming soup, and taking trays of fresh-baked muffins from the oven. And she smiled to herself when she thought about her mother playfully swatting the family's pet Doberman pinscher, Ginger, when the nosy dog got underfoot.

She could almost hear her mother laughing uproariously with her four sisters as they teased and joked with their only brother. Vivian always seemed to be the center of her large family, entertaining them in the various apartments they lived in on Howard and Saratoga and Hopkinson avenues in Bedford-Stuyvesant. No matter how many people were present – including Grandma Leta, her mother-in-law, who lived with the family – Vivian managed to make every one of them feel like a special guest. But providing most of the glamour was Leta herself, who never tired of describing her days of dancing in the chorus of the Ziegfeld Follies, where her sister, Neida Snow, was a featured dancer.

In the midst of her reverie, Lorraine suddenly was enveloped in sadness. As she considered how healthy and strong she felt, how rosy her future looked, how many more years she anticipated living, and the great plans she had for the future, it struck her that she was just a few weeks away from living longer than her mother had.

The difficulty of recalling her mother's death was compounded by the bizarre circumstances surrounding it. Lorraine thought back to her wedding day, when she was 20. But her beautiful wedding gown, the resplendence of the Huntington Townhouse where the event was being held, even the color of her bridesmaids dresses blurred as she remembered the horrifying moment when one of her bridesmaids rushed into the bridal room, where Lorraine was fixing the ribbons on the bouquet she planned to throw to all of her eager single friends.

Her friend's face was ashen, her eyes wild with panic. For a brief moment, Lorraine thought she was going to tell her that the three-tiered wedding cake had fallen on the floor or that someone had had too much to drink and thrown up.

But the news was much worse than anything Lorraine could have imagined. In the midst of the celebration, while standing and speaking with friends, Vivian had suddenly fallen to the floor and died. In her excitement over her only daughter's wedding, she apparently had forgotten to take her medication and suffered a massive heart attack. She was 49 years old.

In one moment, Lorraine's entire world changed. Instead of departing with her new husband for a honeymoon in Quebec, she and John attended her mother's funeral. Great sadness followed, as well as concern for her father, who only a few days before had lived in a bustling household.

Now, with his older son out of the house for many years, with Lorraine a new bride, and with his younger son leaving for the Navy, James was forced to place his mother in a nursing home and face living alone for the first time since he and Vivian had married 32 years before. Although his job as a stationary engineer at Doubleday Publishing Company in Garden City kept him busy, he was a lonely man and it would be many years before Lorraine would see him smile again.

As she stood in her kitchen, flooded with memories, one thought kept going through Lorraine's mind: 49, 49, 49. She was not particularly superstitious, but for years the notion had gnawed at her that somehow that number, that year of her life, would be significant. Flicking away the bothersome idea, she turned her attention to happier thoughts.

She knew that John and their children were planning a big birthday bash for her and that they wanted it to be a reunion of all her relatives, neighbors, and many of the long-lost friends she had known and loved growing up. She already had begun to collect addresses, and she intended to wear a dress that would knock everyone's eyes out.

Life *was* good for Lorraine and she prided herself on consciously appreciating her blessings, of "smelling the roses." She was happy about her job selling real estate and proud of earning a salary. With some of "her own" money, she had recently bought herself a new bicycle and was pleased that after years of procrastinating she had begun a regular exercise program, either walking or bike-riding with her neighbor Roger Ryan.

At that moment, the only things Lorraine had to worry about were the sale of a commercial real estate property to a particularly difficult customer, a broken nail that she planned to have fixed at her regular manicure appointment the next day, thinking up a dinner for that evening, and helping her daughter out with a minor concern.

The day went uneventfully, and as she prepared for bed that night – putting on her nightgown, applying cold cream to her face, brushing her teeth – she reviewed the next day's activities in her mind, setting priorities and thinking about the outfit she'd wear in the evening to one of the many political events she regularly attended with John.

As she climbed into bed, she remembered that she had one more thing to do, something she might not have been so diligent about if she hadn't had fibrocystic breasts and if she hadn't lived on Long Island for so many years. For a brief moment, it occurred to her to skip it, to give herself a breast self-examination in the morning or perhaps the next night. But being a creature of habit, she decided that the vow she had made to herself to perform BSE on the first day of each month – an examination she had been carrying out faithfully for 10 years – must take precedence over her fatigue.

Like many Long Island women, Lorraine was aware of the fact that she lived in a region with an unusually high – even frightening – incidence of breast cancer. A few years earlier, *Newsday*, the Island's only daily newspaper, had run a small article reporting that the incidence of the disease in both Nassau and Suffolk counties was higher than the state's average and that women in Suffolk (where Lorraine lived) had a higher mortality rate.

When she'd read the article, and many articles that followed in other newspapers over the years, Lorraine had been disturbed but not panicked. Though she had been meeting an increasing number of women – many of them in their 30s, 40s, and 50s – who had breast cancer, she still believed in the profile of high-risk women that she'd read. For the most part, she didn't fit it.

Her mother, grandmothers, and cousins never had breast cancer, although she did remember an aunt who'd had the disease. Her first period came late, she gave birth to her children young, and she didn't smoke, drink, or eat high-fat foods. She *had* taken high-estrogen birth control pills, but only for a couple of months. She hadn't taken estrogen-laced hormone replacement therapy. And, except for some dental X-rays, a couple of chest X-rays and mammograms every two years beginning when she was 40, she hadn't been exposed to any large doses of radiation. In the laundry list of risk factors, hers were not considered high.

But that didn't stop her from "playing it safe," performing BSE once a month and having regular mammograms.

In later years, Lorraine would explain her diligence by saying, "I knew I was looking at an epidemic even though no one was calling it that and I knew that in an epidemic no one is safe."

So there she was, exhausted, lying in her cozy bed and giving herself a breast-self examination, when suddenly she felt something unlike any of the familiar "landmarks" she had felt before. Ask any woman who performs BSE and she will tell you that BSE familiarizes a woman with her body in a very particular and intimate way: the contours of the breasts, the shape of the nipples, the little lumps and bumps that were always there and those that are new and demand medical examination.

As she always did during a BSE, Lorraine followed the American Cancer Society's guidelines by placing her right hand behind her head and using the first three fingers of her left hand to palpate her right breast. Starting at the 12 o'clock position on the top of the breast, she slowly moved her fingers in a clockwise direction: 1 o'clock, 2 o'clock, 3 o'clock. When she had rounded the clock, she checked under her arm and, satisfied that nothing had changed since her last BSE, placed her left hand behind her head and began to examine her left breast with the fingers of her right hand. The exam was always the same, month after month, year after year. Clockwise around the breast, check the underarm region, thank God, go to sleep.

And so it went. Twelve o'clock: okay. One o'clock: okay. Two o'clock: okay. Three o'clock: okay. Four o'clock: okay. Five o'clock: okay. But when she got to six o'clock, the very bottom of her left breast, there it was – the unfamiliar something that wasn't supposed to be there.

The room was pitch black. John was already snoring. Lorraine's eyes, which had been closed in semi-sleep, snapped open. "This is not right," she said silently to herself. Resisting panic, she changed her position, confident that the "all clear" mammogram report she had received a few months earlier was "the real truth." But as she felt the spot again, there it was – THE LUMP! Shaking John awake, she cried, "Feel this! What *is* this?" John stirred, turned over, and roused himself.

"You've had a million of these," he said reassuringly. "It's nothing, but you'll call the doctor tomorrow and check it out. Then you'll feel better." It was true, Lorraine thought. She'd felt lots of lumps in her breasts over the years and had had several biopsies to check them out. All of them had been benign, but waiting for the results, she remembered, had taken "a few years off my life."

Lorraine greeted John the next morning with a cheery smile, but as soon as he left for work she ran to the phone to call her radiologist and schedule a mammography.

"But you just had one a few months ago," he told her, "and the results were entirely negative."

"This feels different," Lorraine said, her anxiety rising. The doctor agreed to see her and after palpating the lump agreed to do another screening.

As she waited nervously for the results in the chilly waiting room, still wearing the flimsy gown the technician had given her, Lorraine found herself chanting the mantra she had put out of her thoughts two days before: "49, 49, 49."

When the doctor entered the room, his voice was upbeat but his expression, as Lorraine read it, was grim.

"I think I see a microcalcification in your right breast," he said, "but there's something suspicious in the left breast. We have to check it out."

Quelling a rising sense of panic, Lorraine's words spilled out. "Suspicious! What do you mean suspicious? What does that mean?"

But before the doctor could answer, Lorraine took charge. "Let's do it right away," she said. "This is a big month for me. Business is hectic, I have a million plans, and I'm having a big 50th birthday party!"

A couple of days later, John drove Lorraine to the hospital for the surgery. When the doctor told her the results, both his voice and expression were positive. He had found the microcalcification in the right breast and removed it, and he had removed a fatty lipoma in her left breast.

"You were worried for nothing," the doctor told her.

Lorraine had tried to imagine how she'd react if she were told the lump was malignant. She pictured herself being cool and collected, calmly asking the doctor what would happen next and how she should proceed. In another moment, she pictured herself getting angry, asking the doctor why the lump hadn't been detected in the mammogram she'd had just a few months before. In yet another fantasy, she pictured herself dissolving in tears, feeling completely lost at sea, without a compass or even a star to guide her. But she never imagined how she might react if she were told that the lump was benign.

However, at the sound of the words "You were worried for nothing," Lorraine surprised herself by jumping up from her chair, racing around the doctor's desk, and giving him "the biggest bear hug he'd ever gotten." He laughed. She laughed. And the nurse who was present also laughed and received a big bear hug herself.

Lorraine was so thrilled that she found herself singing the Beatles tune "Good Day Sunshine" in the parking lot on the way to her car. As John turned the key in the ignition, Lorraine was again surprised to find her thoughts going in a completely unanticipated direction. She asked John, instead of going straight home, to take a detour to a party shop a few blocks from their home, where she bought two packages of confetti to throw into the air at her upcoming party.

The days that followed flew by, and suddenly her house and yard were filled with party guests, all offering toasts to Lorraine's health and longevity, all feeling as if they were celebrating something wonderful. Lorraine felt the same and took the opportunity, to everyone's delight, to throw that confetti.

Although still wrapped in bandages and wincing occasionally at a too-tight hug, she spent the day elated to have reached the age of 50 in good health, thrilled that the surgery was over, and thankful beyond thankfulness that she didn't have breast cancer.

It wasn't long before she was back in full swing. She had put the anxiety of the month behind her and, still bandaged, skipped her July 1 breast self-examination. When August 1 rolled around, she resumed her routine and once again felt the lump that had caused her so much dread. She still didn't like the feel of it but reminded herself that her recent mammography screening as well as surgery proved that she had been "worried for nothing." The pathology report said that the tissue the surgeon removed was benign, and that was that.

Nevertheless, as she lay in the dark of her room, Lorraine lectured herself silently, as she often did when she felt nervous. "We're in the 1990s, with the most advanced medicine in the world," she said. "Thank God I'm okay."

That didn't stop her from calling the doctor the next day to tell him that she still didn't like the feel of that 6 o'clock mass. She was surprised when the doctor told her that he hadn't removed *that* mass because "it didn't even show up on the mammogram," but quickly reassured when he added that he thought it was scar tissue left over from previous surgery.

"Come back in six months for your regular checkup," he said. "And stop worrying!"

Finally satisfied that she was really, truly okay, Lorraine plunged back into her busy life with newfound energy. Months went by, and she performed her monthly breast self-examinations with less anxiety. Even though she still felt the lump, her silent lectures abated. She didn't like feeling the "scar tissue," but she was grateful that after all she'd been through it wasn't breast cancer.

As a cold and blustery winter rolled around, she and John decided to take a vacation to the warmer climes of Florida. They visited friends, basked in the sun, ate dinner in wonderful restaurants, and unwound from their busy schedules.

Whenever they ran away to Florida, which was usually when New York was blanketed with snow and it took hours to travel on the Long Island Expressway to a destination that ordinarily took minutes, Lorraine and John talked about moving to the Sunshine State, relocating to the land of palm trees, orange groves, sprawling shopping malls, year-round golf games, and, most of all, sun!

While both of them had deep roots on Long Island, at these moments Lorraine could envision herself forging a new life in what appeared to both of them – on their vacations – to be a less hectic existence.

But on this trip, Lorraine dismissed the idea of relocating. With her children on their own and flourishing in her own job, she felt as if life on Long Island had never been better. She told John that sun was fun but that it wasn't good for them anyway and that she wouldn't be ready to "settle down" for a good 30 or 40 years.

John couldn't have agreed more. While both of them liked the fantasy of moving to Florida, neither of them was eager to give up their active and challenging lives. John not only enjoyed a booming law practice but also for years had been an energetic activist in Long Island politics.

In fact, the Pace brothers – John, Anthony, and Frank – were well known as generous contributors to political campaigns as well as behind-the-scenes forces in shaping many of the policies that made the region's Republican Party the most powerful "machine" in the country. John had been a zone leader for nine years. Anthony had been chairman of the Town of Islip Republican Committee. And Frank, before he left politics, had been a Republican committeeman for nearly a decade.

It was not at all unusual for John and Lorraine to receive special-status invitations to important events sponsored by the most high profile people in political life. While many people are intimidated in the presence of elected officials who are routinely featured on the front page of *The New York Times*, the Paces were on a first-name basis with Senator "Al" D'Amato, Governor "Mario" Cuomo, state House Speaker "Ralph" Marino, and Nassau County Executive "Tom" Gulotta.

At their home in West Islip, John and Lorraine often entertained the politicians and business moguls who played major roles in determining Long Island's fortune. It was a heady life that they doubted a move to Florida could improve upon.

It was also a luxurious life by any standard, although John and Lorraine often laughed about the degree to which they were so "typical." Every day they got up early and went to work, John to his law practice and Lorraine to her real estate job. Most evenings they were busy as well, John attending political meetings and Lorraine spending time with their children and friends.

They also loved spending their weekends going to Broadway shows in Manhattan and dining in many of the finest of the city's million or so restaurants. While they saw their children frequently and talked to them on the phone almost every day, Lorraine and John were enjoying a freedom they hadn't experienced for nearly 30 years.

For Lorraine, there was no more having to think about dinner for five every evening, no more piles of laundry and no more juggling her own pursuits to fit them in with everyone else's schedules. For all the years her children were growing up, Lorraine had been a full-time "hands-on" mother, attending untold numbers of PTA meetings, being a den mother and Brownie leader and carpooling her own and other kids to lessons, dentists, ball games, and the like. But she had also managed to find time to carpool herself to school, taking both day and night classes to earn an associate degree from Suffolk Community College and then a four-year degree in business from Dowling College.

Her imagination enlivened by the world that lay outside her home, she continued her education at Dowling to earn a master's degree in education. While John's salary offered her the opportunity to be a "lady of leisure," spending her days in spas that entice customers with promises of rejuvenation and luxury, she chose to study further for a real estate license at the New York Institute of Technology on Long Island.

Thus armed with three college degrees and a real estate license, Lorraine entertained a variety of enticing job offers. But the lure of the job her son offered her in his Bay Shore real estate business was irresistible, including as it did reasonable hours, decent pay and a short commute. Lorraine found a niche selling commercial buildings and homes, many of which her son John had built.

Lorraine loved the job. She loved her life. She loved Long Island. The annual conversation she usually had with John about relocating to Florida was all but moot.

Toward the end of their vacation, John decided to return to New York a few days early to settle some business affairs. Lorraine stayed on, enjoying her visit and catching up on old times with friends and with her brother Larry, who had traveled from California to see his "big sister."

As she boarded the plane for her return trip to New York, Lorraine had no idea that before she arrived back in the Big Apple, her life would change forever.

Chapter Two

The Undertaker's Warning

Walking down the crowded aisle of the plane, Lorraine found her seat and settled in for the two-and-a-half-hour flight to McArthur Airport in Islip, just 20 minutes from her home. She had picked up a couple of fashion magazines and gossipy tabloids at the Florida airport and anticipated reading about the latest spring colors and the hot scandals on her way back to New York. Within minutes of takeoff, however, her plan went out the window.

Sitting next to her was a handsome man with salt-and-pepper hair who appeared to be in his early or mid-50s. As the plane began its takeoff, he detected Lorraine's nervousness.

"This is my favorite part of the flight," he volunteered.

Lorraine was astonished because taking off and landing were nightmares to her. But she grasped the opportunity to be distracted and asked him why in the world he liked taking off when that was supposed to be the most dangerous part of the flight.

"Because that's when I'm closest to the ground," he explained, "and as long as I'm near the ground, I'm okay."

In spite of her nervousness, Lorraine laughed out loud. "I never thought about that," she said. "And I suppose you like landing too."

"Of course," he said, once again making it apparent that he was full of fun and personality. "That's when I remember all my best jokes!"

Again Lorraine laughed. "Got any jokes now? I could use one!"

And he did. He told her one joke and then another, and she laughed and laughed and laughed. And that was the beginning of a two-and-a-half-hour flight that felt like two and a half minutes to Lorraine.

But it wasn't all jokes. As the flight continued, they discussed many topics. They talked about politics and discovered that they knew many of the same people. They talked about their kids – they both had three – and went on for some time about the high moments of raising kids as well as the war stories. Lorraine told him about her job selling real estate. And, of course, they talked about the weather.

About half way through the flight, after they had been talking nonstop for over an hour, it occurred to Lorraine that she didn't know the man's name and he didn't know hers.

"I'm Lorraine Pace," she announced.

"A pleasure to meet you, Lorraine," he responded. "I'm Arthur Giove."

As they continued chatting, it struck Lorraine that she had told Arthur a lot about herself but knew very little about him.

"What do you do?" she inquired.

"Do you really want to know?" he said.

"Of course," she answered.

"Guess!"

So Lorraine went through the usual laundry list of professions: Lawyer? No. Doctor? No. Teacher? No. Engineer? No. Accountant? No. Businessman? "Well, yes, you could say that."

"What kind of business?" she asked.

"Guess!"

Manufacturing? No. Retail? No. The guesses went on and on.

"I give up," she said.

Arthur lowered his voice to an almost inaudible mumble and said, "Ma'am, I'm your friendly undertaker – also known as a mortician. Actually, I'm a funeral home director and I own three funeral homes on the east end of Long Island."

Lorraine's eyes lit up. "You're kidding!" she exclaimed. "Maybe you know the friend I was just visiting in Florida, Cathleen Chapey – her late husband, Fred, owned the Chapey Funeral Homes in West and East Islip and their two sons are also morticians. You're the third mortician I've spoken to in three days!"

"That's amazing!" Arthur responded, saying that, yes, he knew Fred and his sons.

"I know," Lorraine shot back, adding somewhat cryptically, "I wonder if that means something."

They both laughed at Lorraine's macabre joke, and the next 15 minutes were taken up with undertaker tales, Arthur's firsthand experience and a few hilarious memories that Lorraine shared with him, including one her friend Cathleen Chapey had told her about some mischievous high schoolers who would steal out at night and change the letters on Chapey's Funeral Home, deleting the "C" and blacking out the "eral" in funeral so the sign read "Hapey's Fun Home."

Lorraine laughed so hard while relating this story and Arthur roared so loudly that they were startled to hear the pilot's voice over the public address system announcing that only 15 minutes remained of the flight and thanking them for flying with his airline.

Delving in her pocketbook to find a lipstick and comb, Lorraine turned to her new friend and remarked, "You must like your job – you're such an upbeat person."

She was surprised when Arthur's jovial mood changed and his benevolent expression turned into a gloomy frown.

"I always loved my job, it's true," he said, "because I always felt that I was helping people at a very difficult time in their lives. But now I don't love it because it seems that everything is upside down. It used to be that people died when they got old and that seemed appropriate. Even though a death is always sad, when elderly people die after they've lived their lives and worked and had children and seen life, you have the feeling that this is the way God intended it. But in the past few years, I can't tell you how many young women from the East End of Long Island and the South Fork I've buried who have died of breast cancer. This is not normal. Something is wrong. I warn every woman I meet, no matter how young or old they are, to get a cancer checkup."

Lorraine was so riveted by what Arthur was saying that she barely noticed when the plane bumped to a landing. Suddenly everyone was standing up, grabbing their luggage from the overhead bins, and streaming into the aisles. Things were so hectic that all Lorraine could do was promise Arthur that she'd stay in touch with him and give the lanky six-footer a quick hug.

As she hurried down the aisle and as she stood waiting for John to pick her up, breathing in the brisk winter air of Long Island, her thoughts raced, her mind ablaze with a thought that would haunt her all the way home.

Finally, the thought took the form of a question: "Could it be that the lump I've been feeling in my breast for so many months *is* cancer even though I've been told repeatedly that it's only scar tissue?"

Lying in her bed that night, she tossed restlessly from side to side. The only thing that alleviated her anxiety was the knowledge not only that she had an appointment with her doctor in New York City the next day but also that she had been a vigilant patient all along as a result of her history of fibrocystic breasts and multiple surgeries to remove benign lumps and microcalcifications.

The minute she entered the office and saw her doctor, her words tumbled out.

"I know that the mammograms and sonograms I had were all negative and that the surgery showed nothing," she told him, "but this 6 o'clock lump still bothers me and I just don't think it should be here."

Once again, the doctor examined the lump and reassured her that it was scar tissue. But Lorraine insisted on another mammography. While he didn't seem reluctant to send her for another screening, he did remind her that the test involved a low dosage of radiation and that she had already had three mammograms – with over a dozen views – in that year alone.

He knew, however, that this clinical information and his reassurances were useless. He had known Lorraine for many years and knew her to be unrelentingly persistent.

"Whatever risk is involved," she told him, "I'll sign a paper that I know what the potential dangers are. But I want the mammography!"

A couple of days later she had the test, joking with the technician that "If I don't have breast cancer already, all these mammograms will probably give it to me!"

The results, once again, were negative, but to doubly bolster her confidence, the doctor suggested another sonogram, which in his experience, he said, sometimes detected "something" that mammography failed to pick up. So Lorraine had a sonogram and that, too, was negative.

"What you're feeling is scar tissue," the doctor reassured her.

This time, however, the undertaker's warning was all Lorraine needed to demand that the doctor remove the lump that she had been feeling in her breast in the six-o-clock position for nearly a year.

The doctor didn't exactly argue with her, but he reminded her that the new mammography machines were designed to pick up even the smallest masses and that sonograms augmented their findings and could detect even microscopic masses that mammograms sometimes missed. He told her that the surgery she had had a few months before – and the biopsy – had confirmed that the lump she felt was scar tissue. He urged her not to worry.

Although she had an impulse to scream, Lorraine controlled her rising sense of urgency and, with an edge in her voice, said, "If you don't remove this lump, I'll go to a million doctors until I find someone who will!"

So in March of 1992, a full nine months after Lorraine had first felt that scary lump, the doctor removed it. And under the dense scar tissue, undetected by the mammograms and the sonograms and the previous surgery, was a mass of one and a half centimeters. And yes, it was malignant, as she had somehow – in the deepest recesses of her being – suspected all along.

Lorraine didn't have time to be shattered. Not a minute after giving his diagnosis, the doctor told her that she had to undergo a lumpectomy and the removal of most and perhaps all of the lymph nodes under her arms in order to determine if the cancer had spread. Numb from the news, her head swirled with helter-skelter memories of all the monthly BSE exams she had performed, the numerous treks she had made to doctor after doctor over the previous months, and the test results she had waited for so anxiously.

Lorraine felt anesthetized, as if the part of her brain that ordinarily generates feelings and thoughts had been deadened. John and Lorraine's friend Debra Gorstein held onto her as she got into the car like a sleepwalker. With Debra providing words of optimism and comfort, they drove through the Midtown Tunnel and wended their way in stop-and-start traffic back to West Islip. As John turned into the driveway, Lorraine had a vision of herself throwing the confetti in the air at her 50th birthday party. But she felt nothing.

And she continued to feel nothing when they went out to dinner that evening. The feeling of nothingness continued as she undressed for bed. But as she looked at her breasts in the mirror, the tears started to flow. And they didn't stop. Sitting in her darkened bedroom that evening, all she could do was recite her old mantra: 49, 49, 49.

"I'll be with you soon, Mom," she whispered in despair, "at 50."

A few days later, Lorraine went back into the hospital to undergo an auxiliary dissection of her lymph nodes and a lumpectomy. A week later, she received the results: three of her lymph nodes were found to be cancerous and her doctor told her that she would have to undergo immediate chemotherapy and radiation treatments to try to stop the cancer from spreading further. Lorraine was stunned. Unbelieving. Horrified. Sick at heart. Defeated.

"I'm going to die," she said to herself. "In spite of my suspicions and the care I took to do *everything* right, in spite of my careful BSEs and doctors' visits and living a clean life and believing in God, I'm going to die."

It was a shattering moment. The moment when Lorraine faced her mortality and found that all she had ever heard about people facing death was true. Her entire life raced through her mind: her mother's death on the day of her wedding; the final, Herculean push as she gave birth to her first child; the moment she walked out of her last class in college and realized that she was an independent person. And, again, the blaze of confetti she had thrown in the air with such exuberance only a few months before.

It was one of those existential moments in which she knew that in spite of the people who loved her and believed in her and supported her in every way, she was completely alone. No one but her, she realized, had experienced her mother's death in the same agonizing way that she had, felt the pain and exhilaration of pushing out her first baby, suffered the deep grief she had felt when she learned that her second baby, Jeffrey, had died of hyaline membrane disease.

No one but her had mourned as she did when her father died at the age of 76 , when the vigorous and healthy man she had always known walked into a hospital for a routine test and, not long after, was pronounced dead, possibly, the doctors said, from an allergic reaction to the test's dye. No one but her had sat for weeks and months and years on end in college classes, juggling the needs of her children – and her guilt at being away from them – with her own thirst for knowledge. And no one but her could ever have opened that package of glitzy confetti with the same spirit of celebration or tossed it in the air with such exuberance to thank God for the great gift of what she then believed was her health.

To this day, Lorraine considers these powerful memories as one of the turning points in what would become her new life. Yet, as they coalesced in her consciousness, she realized how little control she – or anyone – had over the great events of their lives.

For a moment, actually for several long moments, she felt on the verge of hysteria, her mind racing with images of the invisible cancer cells in her body multiplying wildly, barreling their way insidiously to distant locations. She remembered the confident tone of her doctor's voice over the past many months, telling her again and again and again that the lump she felt was "nothing." With increasing despair, she wondered how she would ever find – or trust – a doctor to take care of her. Cardiopulmonary resuscitation couldn't save her mother, she thought, and modern medicine can't save me.

Lorraine had once heard the term "runaway anxiety" but she'd had no idea what it meant. Now she was in the throes of it and felt agitated, unstrung, and completely out of control. She jumped up from her bed and started pacing the room, plying herself with the bromides she'd once used to calm her children. "Take a deep breath," she told herself. "Try to relax. Think clearly." At every directive, she felt worse. Flinging herself on the bed again, she started to batter her pillow, screaming at the soft, downy punching bag as if *it* had caused her such grief.

"I hate you!" she cried. "How could you do this to me? *Why* did you do this to me?"

Nothing helped. In her whole life, she had never experienced such hopelessness – or such dread. Running to the bedroom door, she flung it open and screamed into the air: "John, John, where are you?"

But she knew he wasn't there, because just a few minutes before she had told him that she wanted to be alone and, in an effort to be accommodating, he had left the house to do a few errands. Now,

The Undertaker's Warning

panicky at being alone, Lorraine crumpled to the floor like a limp dishrag, immobilized.

For what seemed like a thousand hours, she stayed in the same position, too depleted to shed any more tears or to rail against her cruel fate. As the seconds and minutes went by, she slowly started to stir. From a remote place in her mind, she thought of the title of a book by Richard Farina, the folk singer married to Joan Baez's sister, Mimi, that she remembered from her music-mania days in the late 1960s: "Been Down So Long It Looks Like Up to Me." In spite of herself, she smiled.

In one of those strange connections the mind makes, the thought of the song title served to energize Lorraine. "Hmmm," she mused out loud. "I haven't been down *so* long."

It was a simple thought. Only six words. But it seemed to have a magical effect. Lorraine lifted her head and arose from her catatonic position. But as she walked across the room, the feeling of anxiety seized her once again, literally driving her to reach for the phone and dial a number that was very familiar to her.

"Hello," said the mellow, comforting, baritone voice on the other end of the phone.

"I have breast cancer!" Lorraine wept into the phone. "Why did this happen? What am I supposed to do?"

Amazingly, Father "Tom" Arnao recognized Lorraine immediately, even though he usually talked with her when her voice was lilting

49

and happy. He had been her parish priest for years, as well as a good friend, and she knew that if anyone on earth could help her, it would be her trusted friend. And she was right.

"Lorraine," Father Tom said, "I hear your anger and I hear your grief and you have a right to both. But you're a strong person with a history of fight in you. If you can take this terrible thing that's happened to you and take your anger and do something positive with it, then hopefully a blessing can come out of all your grief."

Father Arnao's voice had a soothing effect on Lorraine. More than that, his words resonated in her, imbuing her with a sense, however tentative, of optimism. She thanked him for his kindness and his wisdom, hung up the phone, and walked calmly to her bathroom. She combed her thick blond hair until it was beauty-salon perfect, splashed cold water on her face, brushed her cheeks with blush, and applied fresh lipstick. She smoothed her blouse, straightened her skirt, and walked serenely into her living room.

As that very moment, John – as if on cue – walked in the front door.

"Where are you going all dolled up?" he kidded her.

"Let's go out," she said. "I just had a little tantrum but I got over it, and now I want some hot tea and a big piece of apple crumb cake with vanilla ice cream!"

And that was it. In the unique way people all over the world are forced to face their own mortality, Lorraine had faced hers. As soon as she told herself that she hadn't been down "so" long, her sense of perspective returned. She was never to lose it again, because with that perspective had come a resolution. Having realized that she was not "in control" of the big things in life, she resolved to be in control of everything that she *could* control.

Her first challenge was to find doctors she could trust, and she set out to do that with a vengeance. After being misdiagnosed for so long, she was aware of the importance of being scrupulously careful in choosing her new doctors. The first people she turned to were the many women she knew who had been diagnosed with breast cancer. To a one, they told her that she had to participate in her own treatment, ask a million questions, risk being considered a "difficult" patient, and never be shy about suggesting a new or alternative treatment she had read or heard about.

"Never settle," one of her friends told her. "If you're not getting the kind of treatment you think you deserve, don't hesitate for one second to look for another doctor, even if you have to do it a dozen times."

Lorraine knew this only too well, but hearing it from "seasoned" cancer patients helped to reinforce her own conviction that, above all, she should trust her instincts and, as her friend told her, "never settle."

Another friend for whom she had tremendous respect recommended an oncologist, Dr. Michael Feinstein, whose office was in Plainview. And a physician friend from California advised her to call the American College of Radiology to find out who was certified in radiation oncology in Suffolk County. That is how she discovered Dr. Allen G. Meek, a radiation oncologist from the Department of Radiation Oncology at University Hospital and Medical Center at Stony Brook – the only department in the specialty that was certified in Suffolk County at the time.

Lorraine didn't go for her first visits to these two doctors wearing boxing gloves, but both of them knew the minute they met her that she meant business. And, as sometimes happens, they liked that. No matter how many questions she asked, they took the time to answer them. No matter how many anxieties she expressed, they had the patience to allay them. If it is true, as some studies have indicated, that combative patients fare better than passive patients, then Lorraine appeared to be one woman who – with the help of chemotherapy and radiation – would intimidate her cancer cells out of existence.

In retrospect, Lorraine would attribute her fighting spirit to a heartbreaking episode in her life that, she said, "was a dress rehearsal for my fight against breast cancer."

Nearly 20 years before she was diagnosed, when she was 31 and caring for her three young children, one of them an infant, Lorraine's older brother Ronald, who was recently divorced, returned from Hawaii to live in West Islip with his father and his two teenage children, Jerry and Laura Jane, who he had agreed to care for full time. A short time later, after Ronald moved with the children into a rented home in Bay Shore, he was stricken with a severe stroke that left him in a coma. Lorraine took over the care of her nephew and soon noticed that the 14-year-old, who had cerebral palsy, was experiencing both difficulty walking and crashing headaches.

The boy's pediatrician attributed his unsteady gait to the cerebral palsy and told Lorraine that the headaches were probably because he needed eyeglasses. But Lorraine did her own research and suspected that his condition was significantly worse than the doctor had pronounced. Sure enough, the ophthalmologist detected a much graver problem in Jerry: a brain tumor that was pressing on the teenager's optic nerve. Without immediate surgery, he said, the boy had a poor chance of survival.

As a de facto surrogate parent, Lorraine acted immediately, giving permission to the neurosurgeon to remove the rapidly- growing tumor, which had ballooned to the size of a grapefruit at the base of Jerry's brain. The young man recovered from his surgery but when he was 40, he suffered a severe seizure and was admitted to a nursing home, at the same age his father was when he was felled by a stroke and also admitted to a long-term care facility. In a strange and tragic coincidence, Lorraine lost both her father and oldest brother in 1986, Ronald at the age of 53, and the patriarch of their once flourishing family three months later, at the age of 76.

These experiences stayed with Lorraine, convincing her that arming oneself with knowledge, trusting one's instincts, pursuing a proper diagnosis in spite of the discouragement of this or that "expert," and being a strong advocate were essential ingredients in facing illness – any illness. Little did she suspect that she would bring all of these qualities to bear in her fight against breast cancer.

In the days and weeks following her surgery, Lorraine was constantly busy going to her new doctors, reading everything she could get her hands on, talking to anyone and everyone who offered advice, and trying to keep herself from the panic and despair she had experienced when she crumpled to the floor.

That wasn't easy. She couldn't help picturing how sick she'd feel and how ravaged she'd look from her chemotherapy treatments and, worse, imagining that the cancer cells were spreading out of control. She feared that her own death, unlike her mother's, which had been sudden, would be protracted and painful.

Indeed, the treatments were, as Lorraine said in retrospect, "not easy." She lost a lot of her luxuriant blonde hair, experienced nausea and vomiting, and felt sick for days on end. On numerous occasions, she thought about the rituals of the ancient cultures she had studied in school in which aged or dying people, in order to spare their families the sight or burden of their prolonged deaths, simply wended their way to a remote mountaintop or the edge of the ocean in order to lie down and die in peace.

There were moments she felt on the verge of a nervous breakdown. To combat the feelings, she indulged in her drug of choice: bike-riding with her friend and neighbor Roger Ryan. With an uncanny knack for diverting Lorraine's attention, Roger kept their conversations focused on living in the moment, making sure that the time they spent together always focused on bike talk: tire treads and mileage, gear shifts and reflectors, helmets and wind jackets. Occasionally he steered the talk to the weather or to the beautiful spring flowers that were just beginning to emerge.

Throughout her treatments, additional rays of light appeared to Lorraine in the ongoing encouragement she received from Father Arnao. She talked about his help with her friends, often citing the blessing Father Tom had bestowed on Lorraine and John's house with a prayer and a sprinkling of holy water, remarking with his typical humor: "If I'd known your home was so big, I'd have brought a hose!"

And many cancer patients lent their support as well, particularly one woman who told Lorraine, "Today, more people are *living* with cancer than *dying* from it."

Nevertheless, Lorraine didn't like the way she looked. She didn't recognize her personality. She hated the way she felt. She railed against God. She wept.

But she went on.

And then, as suddenly as the nightmare of her diagnosis was pronounced and as arduous as her treatments were, they were all gone. She was okay. The frightening follow-up tests revealed that she was "clear" of cancer, that *all she would have to do* was to be vigilant about having regular checkups.

"That's all I have to do?" she asked her doctors? "Just keep careful tabs on myself?"

That was it, they said, and sent her off to live her life.

But keeping tabs on cancer was different than keeping tabs on the other things that had given Lorraine anxiety in her life. When her oldest son, John, had a strep throat and penicillin cured it, there were no tabs to keep. When her daughter, Lisa, had a facial cyst removed, there were no tabs to keep. When her youngest son, Greg, got mononucleosis, there were no tabs to keep.

"Keeping tabs" on cancer was another story. How can I ever know, Lorraine thought to herself – and asked her doctors – if that innocent sniffle or that sore back or that bad headache is simply what it seems to be and not those virulent cancer cells inflicting their killer instincts on other parts of my body?

When she found a "lump" on her foot, she feared the worst. "Hmmm," the podiatrist said, "we can remove this if you want."

"If I *want*?" cried Lorraine. "What choice is there when you have a malignant lump?!"

"Oh dear, no wonder you're so upset," the doctor responded. "My dear, dear lady, all you have here is a bunion!"

Lorraine was thrilled that the lump was a bunion, but when she asked her other doctors how she would know if the cancer had spread, all they could say was: "We'll keep a close watch."

No one's fool, Lorraine interpreted those answers as: "We don't know."

And so, life went on for Lorraine, as it did – and it does – for millions upon millions of cancer patients in the United States. But during the months of her treatment and, before that, when she was trying to learn everything she could about breast cancer, she read about things that mystified and infuriated her.

Her most persistent question was: Why, in the most powerful and medically advanced country in the world, has the War on Cancer that President Richard Nixon proclaimed in 1971 been lost? And why does breast cancer seem to be the biggest loser?

In 1960, Lorraine had learned, 1 out of every 20 women got breast cancer. In 1980, that incidence had climbed precipitously, to 1 in 14. In 1990, it was 1 in 9. And Lorraine suspected that on Long Island it was probably 1 in 8.

Just as disturbing was the fact that in the United States, 182,000 women were diagnosed with breast cancer every year and 46,000 died of the disease.

These statistics angered Lorraine. And it bothered and angered her that it was so difficult for her and other women to find doctors they could trust and rely on. And that the radiation and chemotherapy treatments she received were so similar to – and sometimes exactly the same as – the treatments that women with breast cancer had received decades before.

But the harshest lessons she learned – and the most demoralizing – were about being a cancer patient.

While her husband and children and good friends rallied around her with support and encouragement, one of the most painful realities to her was that there were still many people in the early 1990s who considered cancer patients "contagious." Many of the people she considered her extended family – a few colleagues at work and in her political circle, and especially her brothers-in-law and their wives – spoke of cancer as "The Big C" and seemed to regard it as a virtual death sentence.

Lorraine tried to understand – and rationalize – why they distanced themselves from her, but she didn't get it. "Am I that unacceptable?" she wondered. "Have I changed the way I treat my friends or relatives or how I feel about them?"

Of course she was not unacceptable, and, if anything, she felt and expressed the deepest gratitude toward the people who were simply nice to her when she was going through the worst phases of her treatment. But that didn't lessen the hurt she felt when so many people looked at or spoke to her as if she were contaminated.

Ultimately she came to understand their reactions. Just as she had seen people at wakes and Shiva calls say nothing or the wrong thing, she came to realize that death scared most people, rendering them literally lost for words. That is exactly the way most of the people she encountered reacted when someone they knew – including her – was diagnosed with cancer. It was a bittersweet insight, but by this time Lorraine was accustomed to facing hard realities.

Besides, she was discovering a whole new world of extraordinary people who, like her, had been blindsided by cancer. Rather than staying away, they called her with offers of help and advice, invited her to join support groups, shared resources, and introduced her to the generally optimistic world of cancer survivors.

As she began to speak more openly about her condition and drive to support-group meetings that were 20 or 30 or 40 minutes from her home, she realized that the population of cancer patients she was now a part of was more widespread than she had ever imagined. The realization shocked but also encouraged her. The people she met were not dying – they were living! They had not capitulated to their condition – they were fighting it!

They also were starting to ask questions that demanded answers: *Why* were so many women stricken with the disease? *Why* was there such a disproportionate incidence of breast cancer on Long Island? *Why* was it more common here than in New York City and its boroughs, including Queens and Brooklyn, or in nearby Westchester County?

There were no answers. But the questions proliferated, fueled by newspaper articles that questioned *what* role the environment played, *when* answers from the medical and science communities would be forthcoming, *where* those answers would be published or aired, *how* those answers would translate into better treatments or a cure, and *who*, exactly, would find the answer to the scourge that was afflicting the women of Long Island – and the country – in such frightening numbers.

Lorraine listened to and absorbed the enormity of the breast cancer problem on Long Island. She witnessed women in their 20s weep with grief as they recounted the moment they felt a lump in one of their breasts and went blithely to their doctors without a care in the world, only to find that they had cancer.

She heard women in their 30s and 40s who thought they were in "excellent" health and were enjoying their careers as mothers or in business or as professors and attorneys and physicians describe how breast cancer had devastated their lives, plunged them into deep depression, and made them fear every minute of every day.

She heard the laments of women in their 50s and 60s and 70s tell of their horror at discovering that they had breast cancer and describing the difficulty in finding support and encouragement and hope – or even information! And also of the "second-class" treatment they received because, as one 71-year-old woman told her, "They think we should be philosophical about accepting death."

She heard stories of the toll that breast cancer took on the lives of women whose husbands found them sexually unappealing after breast cancer surgery, of boyfriends who abandoned them, of children who didn't know what to do or say.

She heard of brusque and even sadistic doctors who spoke to patients with less humanity than they spoke to deli employees and of robotic hospital technicians who administered radiation and chemotherapy to patients they treated like inanimate objects.

She cried for these people and she cried with them. But in between her tears, Lorraine was obsessed with one question: Why? She had no answer, but the question haunted her every day.

On the positive side, the new relationships she was forging made her realize that there *was* life after cancer, that the big C, for many people, meant Coping and Caring and Conquest.

And, although her chemotherapy treatments were arduous and her participation in the support groups deeply affecting, it wouldn't be long before Lorraine recovered her gregarious personality and added one more C to that list: Crusade.

Chapter Three

Elmer Gantry

Movie fans of the 1970s, '80s, and '90s flocked to films that featured Robert De Niro, Harrison Ford, Matt Damon, Brad Pitt, and Leonardo DiCaprio. But in the '50s and '60s, screen idols like Marlon Brando, Kirk Douglas, Montgomery Clift, and Burt Lancaster were all the rage.

In 1960, a year before she was married, Lorraine went to see "Elmer Gantry" and was transfixed by Burt Lancaster's performance. Something about the charming, itinerant Gantry captured her imagination. The high and mighty in Hollywood agreed with her and millions of other moviegoers who viewed the adaptation of Sinclair Lewis's 1927 novel and awarded Lancaster an Academy Award for his riveting performance.

Gantry was a fake – a con man, gambler, drunkard, and womanizer who mesmerized people with his charisma, accusing them with his fiery revivalist preaching of being sinners while all along he was a sinner himself.

The end of the story shows Gantry being exposed as a fraud by a former lover who blackmails him with tawdry photographs of their trysts. His most impassioned fans become his most ardent detractors, and Gantry is ultimately discredited and ruined.

For some reason, Lorraine's experience with breast cancer evoked memories of the phony preacher. Looking back, she figured out that it was the contradiction in his character – the good guy who was really a bad guy – that she was beginning to see in the breast cancer picture: politicians who claimed to have the public's interest at heart but avoided addressing the scourge of the disease on Long Island; newspaper people who wrote about aerobics and housing starts but failed to investigate possible environmental links to the disease; even some of the "professionals" who administered her chemotherapy and radiation treatments, laughing and telling jokes while she sat waiting for treatment for unconscionable lengths of time in uncomfortable and cold rooms before they administered what she considered poison into her veins.

Something was very wrong, she believed: the "good guys" weren't paying attention. She felt as if a gigantic jigsaw puzzle was waiting to be pieced together but that with few but notable exceptions, most of the people who were in the position to fit the pieces together were asleep on the job.

Ironically, she didn't have to travel to a library, read *The Wall Street Journal*, or attend a seminar to find the puzzle's first piece. All she had to do was take a walk.

In the days before she had surgery, as well as during the most arduous days of her chemotherapy, one of the only things that made her feel better was walking through her neighborhood, breathing the air and chitchatting with neighbors. To her astonishment – and dismay – she learned that in an eight-block radius of her home over 20 women had been diagnosed with breast cancer. The "something" that she felt was wrong was a very big something.

It was the next piece of the puzzle that confirmed her suspicions. One day she noticed employees from the Suffolk County Water Authority working on her street. At the time she didn't think anything of it, but when they returned two more times, Lorraine – never a retiring wallflower – walked out of her house and approached one of the workers.

"What are you doing?"she asked him.

"Blowing out the system," he responded. "Water doesn't circulate as well on dead-end streets as it does in the middle of the block."

The man's voice had a flat, dry, "Just the facts, Ma'am" tone. But his seemingly unremarkable words triggered a remarkable Aha! in Lorraine. With mathematical precision, she immediately computed the two pieces of information she had recently learned: that more than 20 women with breast cancer lived on or near dead-end streets near the Great South Bay and that water on dead-end streets became stagnant because it didn't circulate well.

So stagnant, in fact, that it required paid public employees to periodically "blow out" the system. In an instant, she realized that this *might* be the "something" that explained (or at least was a part of) Long Island's high incidence of breast cancer.

"After all," she thought to herself, "my tap water is filthy and cloudy and so, probably, is the tap water of my neighbors.

Could there be a connection between my filthy tap water, laced as it is with a sediment of heavy metals, and my breast cancer and theirs?"

She was excited by her theory but at the same time insecure about it. She didn't want to believe that the water she and her husband and children and neighbors had been drinking was slowly poisoning them and, worse, causing cancer. In her heart, she hoped that John would tell her she was way off track. But he didn't. He also was looking for answers but he advised Lorraine to "go slow," telling her that she had to have more "proof" and that more important people than her or their neighbors needed to present her theory to the public.

Lorraine was at a loss, wanting to scream her suspicions to the world but aware that a housewife from western Suffolk County on Long Island had little chance of making a case that would be regarded with any degree of seriousness by anyone with the ability to investigate her claims. In other words, anyone in power.

Fate, however, intervened in the form of a *Newsday* article. The seventh-largest daily in the nation, the newspaper had been steadfastly remiss in reporting the escalating incidence of breast cancer cases on Long Island and in exploring this fact's possible relationship to the environment. While the paper's main science reporter had written a number of articles about the disease, most of them echoed "standard" medical system misinformation. They also failed to convey the deep anxiety of Long Island women about the clusters of breast cancer cases that, with increasing frequency, were appearing in residential neighborhoods, schools, and office buildings.

Before Lorraine got breast cancer in 1992, only *The Women's Record* (*TWR*), a small newspaper based on the North Shore of Long Island, had consistently addressed all aspects of the breast cancer problem – clinical, psychological, social, political, and environmental. Although the paper's circulation was modest by any measure, it was mailed to the shakers and movers in the region, including politicians, educators, and members of the medical community – and many of them were beginning to take notice.

Among the many dozens of articles about the disease that had appeared in the paper since 1985 were those discussing the possible relationship of environment to breast cancer, explaining that Long Island's sole-source aquifer system, a closed system of water circulation – much like the body's circulatory system – failed to offer residents an auxiliary source of drinking or bathing water, such as lake runoffs or reservoirs, that other areas of the country count on when their water systems become polluted.

Until the mid-1940s, Long Island was primarily a farming community, its water pure. But when thousands upon thousands of servicemen came back from World War II, the lure of affordable housing offered by the sprawling Levittown housing complex was irresistible. It was not long before major aerospace and other industries followed and with them millions of tons of waste byproducts that permeated the soil and inevitably found their way into the water system.

During these years, children playfully ran after the trucks spraying DDT to kill mosquitoes, laughing when they got lost in the pesticide's fog. The "miracle chemical" was sprayed on vegetables that were served each evening at the dinner table, on cattle from which steaks, roasts, and hamburgers were made, on cotton that became articles of clothing, and on children themselves to "prevent" the blight of polio.

Over the next couple of decades, the population of Nassau and Suffolk counties nearly tripled, and the population's interest in nature and health gave rise to an increasing number of organic gardeners and conservation clubs. The first legal action against DDT began in 1957 when 12 activists lodged the first public lawsuit against the insecticide in response to a huge federal- and state-directed spray campaign against the gypsy moth. Nearly 400,000 gallons of the chemical was sprayed on Long Island, quadruple the amount sprayed in neighboring areas such as Queens or Westchester County.

Four years later, Rachel Carson, the trailblazing author of *Silent Spring* and a breast cancer patient herself, described the fatal effects of pesticides on birds, fiddler crabs, and, she suspected, human beings.

A second lawsuit against DDT, instituted in 1966 by the Brookhaven Town Natural Resources Committee, convinced the judge in the case to suspend Suffolk County's use of the chemical. In 1972, DDT was banned nationally, but the ban did nothing to stop the chemical's breakdown products, such as DDE, from continuing to contaminate the environment or from being increasingly implicated in human ills by science experts.

These were the years in which plastic products were developed and proliferated in industry and household use, spewing forth invisible and toxic PCBs, which, carried on the wind, found their way to wildlife, snow, breast milk, and human skin.

These also were the years in which radiation – "the miracle treatment" – was used routinely in high and unregulated doses on everything from acne to the thymus glands of thousands of babies, many of them female, who science then believed were dying suddenly because of the gland's enlargement.

And these were the years when doctors advertised their favorite cigarette brands on TV. Indeed, these were times when there was simply *no* association between human health and environmental toxins.

We now know that environmental hazards exist throughout the country and that in many cases they have contaminated the soil and the water. But on Long Island, unlike in other parts of the country, there is no getting rid of them. Once they reach the water, they stay there – decade after decade after decade.

Nearly 25 years after the concerns of the early activists on Long Island impelled them to take action against environmental pollutants, the same anxiety prevailed. Several of *TWR*'s articles challenged the design of a study about breast cancer on Long Island, asking why sources of drinking water and pesticides had not been included. The study had been undertaken in 1985, a collaborative effort that included the New York State Department of Health, the health departments of Nassau and Suffolk counties, and the State University at Stony Brook in Suffolk County.

As a result, the design of the study had been changed, but too late for the 1990 press conference at Stony Brook University, held upon publication of the final report of the study.

A little more than a year before she got breast cancer, Lorraine had read about the study's conclusions in *Newsday*. Two major factors, the study said, accounted for the high incidence of the disease on Long Island: a great number of women in high-income brackets (supposedly, one "risk factor") and a large number of Jewish residents (who seemed to have a disproportionate incidence of the disease).

Other factors included having children late in life or not at all, menstruating early, eating a high-fat diet, and taking high-dose birth control pills, all which were thought to heighten cancer risk because they increased a woman's lifetime exposure to the hormone estrogen.

Long Island's women were not happy with these conclusions, not only because they suspected other factors at work but also because the report made it sound as if responsibility for the disease lay with the women themselves!

Lorraine hadn't read *The Women's Record*'s articles over the years, but she did read the column this writer wrote in response to the study, which concluded, "Long Island doesn't have more wealth than Beverly Hills or Shaker Heights and we don't have more Jewish women than Miami Beach or Israel – we just have more breast cancer!"

That made sense to Lorraine, and she filed the article away. At the time, her only thought was "There's more to this problem than meets the eye." But in the busyness of her life she relegated that thought to the back of her mind.

However, when she became a breast cancer patient in 1992 and began her search for answers, the article came back to her when she read a small notice in *Newsday* advertising a May 11 hearing on breast cancer that was being sponsored by Senator Alfonse D'Amato, who had begun to demand federal intervention to review the Long Island Breast Cancer Study's conclusions. It was only a couple of weeks after her surgery and before her chemotherapy treatments had started that Lorraine joined over 250 other interested people at the hearing, held at the Nassau Academy of Medicine.

Elmer Gantry

"Women want to know: Why me? Why now? Why on Long Island? And why in certain pockets of Long Island?" the director of Cancer Care, Harriet Orenstein, asked the panel's four representatives from the Centers for Disease Control and Prevention (CDC) in Atlanta. In over two hours of emotional testimony, speaker after speaker said essentially the same thing: The rate of breast cancer on Long Island is not "normal" and we want you to *do something* about it – specifically, review the study and admit that clusters exist.

Lorraine was accompanied by a friend who also had breast cancer. As they stood patiently in line, waiting for their turns at the microphone, both of them noticed that the CDC panel members were listening to the speakers with their eyes glazed over and that their answers were both patronizing and uninformative. They seemed to be infuriated when one woman finally made it to the microphone and read a published report revealing that Long Island had 139 past and present toxic waste sites and 80 manufacturing facilities that had reported releasing 43 million pounds of 51 toxic chemicals into the environment in one year – only to have a CDC panelist respond that environmental factors had "no known role" in the induction or promotion of cancer.

"Elmer Gantrys," Lorraine said to herself, invoking the image of the good guys who weren't good guys at all.

Not wanting to be on the receiving end of that kind of insulting behavior, she thought about stepping away from the microphone and taking her seat in the audience. But when another women was dismissed out of hand by an expert who told her that Long Island's high incidence of breast cancer was the result of "established risk factors" and "non-environmental causes," Lorraine was furious and resolved to stay in the ever-shortening line.

Just as the forum was drawing to a close, Lorraine stepped up to the mike. The moderator, having received a number of bashing questions, was clearly looking for a moderate voice and Lorraine appeared to be the person he was looking for.

Dressed in a stunning hot-pink suit, her blonde wavy hair just so, and appearing as Mrs. Middle-Class America who would not or could not possibly pose a challenging question, she evoked some welcoming smiles from the embattled panel.

"Yes, Ma'am," the moderator said. "State your name and please ask us your question."

Prepared as she was, Lorraine was still somewhat flustered to finally have the floor. But in her mind – and in bed at night, in her car, in her kitchen, in all of the conversations she had had with her breast cancer compatriots and neighbors and in her talks with the Suffolk County Water Authority worker outside her door – she had rehearsed her question exhaustively.

"Thank you for allowing me to speak," she said in her sweet, lilting, upbeat voice. "This is my question."

Instead of her question, however, Lorraine kept the panel and the audience waiting impatiently as she leaned over to fish for something in her roomy handbag. As the moderator and panel rolled their eyes and fidgeted, Lorraine continued to fish.

Finally, she stood back up and smiled. "I'm sorry for the delay, but I thought this was important." Holding up a large bottle of filthy tap water for the entire forum to behold, she made her case.

"This is my tap water," she said. "This is the water that my children and I and my husband and all of my neighbors have been drinking for many, many years. This is not clean water. It is dirty water. It doesn't taste good. And, as you can see, it doesn't look good. And just recently, some workers from the Suffolk County Water Authority were working on my street and they told me that water doesn't circulate as well on dead-end streets as it does in the middle of the block. I live on a dead-end street and so do a lot of other women – 20 of them in my neighborhood have breast cancer – and the majority of them live on a dead-end too!"

At these words, an audible gasp arose from the audience and Lorraine, slightly flustered, paused to allow the panel to digest her dramatic – and alarming – statement. The panel sat stupefied, clearly unprepared for the hardball statement that had been hurled at them from such an unlikely source.

Regaining her composure, Lorraine continued. "So these are my questions: "I watched my diet and went for mammograms regularly, so why did I get breast cancer? What is in my water? And is this horrible-looking stuff toxic? And is there a connection between my breast cancer and my tap water and the heavy metals in its sediment?"

As Lorraine focused her eyes on each member of the panel, she could see that the scientists had the same look on their faces as her childhood friends in Brooklyn had when they played "Statue" – dumbstruck, unresponsive, frozen. One of them mumbled something about there being "no evidence" that drinking water and breast cancer were related.

But when Dr. Nancy Lee, one of the CDC's experts, was pressed by the audience for a time limit for the agency's report and responded by saying that it would be ready "within six months," a tiny spark of awareness began to take shape in Lorraine's consciousness – a spark that would soon become a bonfire. In six months, while nothing was being done, she wondered, how many more women would be diagnosed with breast cancer?

Her musing was short-lived. The sight of the murky brownish tap water had sent a chill through the audience and, within minutes, people rushed up to Lorraine, wanting to get a closer look and wincing when they did. Reporters surrounded her, plying her with questions: "When did you discover this?" "Did you have the water tested in a lab?" "Does anyone else in your family have cancer?" "Do you accept the answer you got, that there's no connection between your water and cancer?"

Although her answer to the last question was not published, she told the reporter, "No – I can't accept *anything* until I and every woman on Long Island knows why we're getting breast cancer."

The next day, *Newsday*'s front-page article about the forum featured a photo of Lorraine holding her jar of dirty tap water. The enigma of breast cancer on Long Island may have been a million-piece jigsaw puzzle, but once the CDC conference ended Lorraine knew that she might have stumbled onto a major piece of it. All she had to do, she thought, was present this and perhaps other pieces of the puzzle to the medical and science experts who had the power to put them all together and finally make sense of what she continued to call a "terrifying epidemic."

Her optimism didn't last long. Her appearance at the conference had been powerful, and *Newsday*'s front-page article initially generated intense interest in the possible relationship between the horrible-looking drinking water and the horrific incidence of breast cancer. But after a few days, the enthusiasm and curiosity that had greeted her remarks seemed to vanish and all she was left with was her jar of murky tap water.

Actually, that's not *all* she was left with. There was still the image of Elmer Gantry, gallivanting throughout the country accusing naïvely believing people that he was the expert on sin when, in fact, he was its embodiment. While she didn't believe that the scientists on the CDC panel were sinners, at least in the literal meaning of the word, she did think they were wrong when they said there was "no evidence" that environmental pollutants were related to cancer.

She remembered reading about the long battle that a young upstate New York housewife, Lois Gibbs, had waged against both government officials and science experts when she tried to convince them that the raft of miscarriages, neurological disorders and cancer her neighbors suffered from and often succumbed to were related to the toxic chemicals that the Hooker Chemical Company had dumped into the soil – and underneath the elementary school – in Love Canal. Ultimately, Lorraine recalled, the federal government paid to relocate every member of that community, without ever admitting that their diseases were related to the effect of the chemicals.

She thought about the epidemiologist from the Midwest who found what appeared to be a chilling relationship between childhood leukemia and electromagnetic fields from overhead power lines – and the subsequent apparently organized campaign to discredit her. She read with increasing fascination about a case in Woburn, Massachusetts, in which parents attributed their children's leukemia to the carcinogenic toxins that spewed unchecked and unmonitored from a nearby industry and had hired a lawyer to represent them.

In all of these cases, Lorraine noted, the common denominators were a unified lack of accountability from the powers-that-be, a unified contempt for the questions that regular people like her were posing, and a unified resistance to even considering the validity of their claims.

In that respect, she knew she was in good company and never for a moment considered that *all* she had going for her was a jar of murky tap water or the mental image of Elmer Gantry. What was not visible to the outside world was abundantly clear to Lorraine. It was a quality that arose from deep within her, took shape as the days elapsed, and, ironically, was spurred on by the very resistance she encountered.

That quality was resolve. Steady resolve. Firm resolve. Fierce resolve.

Up to this point, Lorraine's life had not been wildly out of the ordinary – with notable exceptions such as her mother dying on her wedding day and getting breast cancer in the prime of her life. The cancer – unfortunately common, as it was and is – made her think not how typical her experience was but how unique.

All at once she began to appreciate that no one in the more than six billion people in the world had her own peculiar fingerprints, her singular configuration of DNA molecules, her own particular take on the world. The thought enlivened her.

While she hadn't grown up in a traveling circus, where riding elephants and swinging from high-wire trapezes are everyday events, or been raised by a naturalist in a jungle setting with apes for siblings, her Brooklyn upbringing had made her tough and her adult accomplishments had made her appreciate the value of sticking with a goal through thick and thin. Now, her mission clear, she would call upon those qualities in her quest for answers.

"I would have been thrilled and elated if someone had told me, had shown me, that my suspicions had no foundation," she said. "But that wasn't the case. It was too late for me, but I have a daughter and my friends have daughters and granddaughters. All I could think of was the next generation and trying to get answers that might save them the horror of being diagnosed with this savage disease."

What to do? What to do? What to do? This question consumed practically every minute of Lorraine's day. She knew she had to do *something*. But what? Sipping tea in her elegant kitchen, she looked at the bottle of murky tap water she kept on the sink as a reminder that grave threats can often be found in the midst of great beauty.

She already had bought a new water filter and was considering ordering one of the brands of spring water that had become so popular on Long Island, but she had placed the bottle on the kitchen counter as a bitter reminder – a symbol – of her breast cancer. As she gazed absently at the bottle, her mind started to wander.

Maybe this is just a fluke. After all, most Long Island women don't live on the water on dead-end streets. I wonder if breast cancer is as common in the rest of West Islip as it is in my neighborhood. I guess I'll never know because I could never walk down every block in town and knock on every door and ask people if they have cancer. I know there are clusters of breast cancer all over Long Island, but the experts say there's no such thing as a cluster. Who am I to challenge the experts? What can I do?

As Lorraine ruminated, a thought slowly entered her mind. Like many revolutionary ideas, it didn't take long to crystallize. Within 15 minutes she had a plan. Scribbling her ideas on a notepad, she grew more and more excited at the prospect of translating her idea into action.

But something was still missing. Tapping her pencil on the table, she searched for the theme of her plan, one simple phrase that would tie it up in a neat, comprehensible package. She bit the tip of her pencil, got up and walked over to her kitchen window, sat back down and took a deep breath.

"Damn," she mumbled to herself. "What am I trying to say?"

And then, like the proverbial light bulb, it came to her. On the top of the pad she scrawled: "No questions, no answers!"

"That's it!" she exclaimed out loud as she jumped from her chair in excitement. "Questions! Oh my God, I have a million questions!"

Most of them started with "why": Why did I get breast cancer? Why do so many of my neighbors have breast cancer? Why do so many women on Long Island have breast cancer? Why do I think I'm living in a "cluster" of breast cancer but none of the experts agree? Why do so many women I know with the disease live near the water? But there was also a "how": How can I prove there's a cluster and that it might be related to our drinking water?"

Thus armed with her "million" questions, Lorraine suddenly visualized her entire town and the untold numbers of women she had never met but somehow suspected had suffered silently, as she had, with a breast cancer diagnosis.

"What if the cluster I think exists in my water's-edge part of West Islip doesn't exist in our whole town?" she wondered. "I'll need a map of the place to ever know the answer!"

Within seconds, her plan was born: to get a map of West Islip and – no matter how long it took – find out the breast cancer history of families in her entire community, the better to establish if her suspicions were true, that a cluster of breast cancer cases in West Islip was somehow related to living near the water.

It was an ambitious plan, immensely more complicated than she imagined as she sat in her kitchen that day. And it was an unprecedented plan. No person – certainly not a middle-aged housewife with an utter lack of scientific training – had ever undertaken a community-wide epidemiological cancer study. In fact, no scientific institution had ever conducted such a study!

Lorraine's lack of sophistication about science matters was on her side. The idea was so pure, so simple and seemingly doable that the complexity of data collection and analysis, publicity and finances and rounding up assistance from a variety of people and places hadn't even occurred to her. She was not thinking about her plan in terms of the long journey it would turn out to be. The only thing she had in mind was the first step – the map.

Within minutes she was on the phone to her friend Michael LoGrande, who she and John knew from their years of socializing and attending Republican Party meetings.

Lorraine often kidded Michael, calling him a teddy bear because of his slightly paunchy middle and his huggableness, and she considered him an honorable and trustworthy person.

But the call she made to his office wasn't social. Michael was the powerful chief executive officer of the Suffolk County Water Authority. When Lorraine told him her idea, she was thrilled that he seemed to support it. He explained that his secretary had died of breast cancer in 1987 and he remembered how mystified she had been that she and so many other women in the region were suffering from the disease.

"But you can't do this alone," LoGrande warned her. "You need some experts on your side." He suggested that she call a few people he thought would be important for the plan to work and offered to set up a meeting "when you're ready."

The first person Lorraine called was her oncologist, Dr. Michael Feinstein, pausing before she hit the last number to reflect on the frightening fact that she knew his number by heart. From the moment she met him, she had felt an immediate bond, sensing that the soft-spoken, portly, balding physician, who she guessed was in his late 50s, cared deeply about his patients. It was apparent to her that he had many years left to practice, so she was surprised when he told her that he was thinking of retiring and that one of the reasons was because he was so upset by the great numbers of young women he was treating for breast cancer.

When he answered her call, the doctor told her that he had read the *Newsday* article that featured her holding the by-now-famous jar of murky water and that he was impressed. But Lorraine atypically skipped the social niceties and blurted out her mission.

"I want to find out why so many women are getting breast cancer on Long Island," she said, her words tumbling out in an unbroken stream. "To ask all the questions I've been asking all along but no one has been answering. So I have a plan to develop a questionnaire that asks all the women – actually all the people in West Islip – the right questions and I'm getting a map and planning to…"

"Whoa!" Dr. Feinstein interrupted her. "I think it's a great idea. How can I help you?"

"Well, I don't know anything about asking the right medical or scientific questions," Lorraine said. "And they have to be right so that no one can say that an uppity housewife who didn't know what she was talking about put together some crazy questionnaire that doesn't mean anything."

"You've got it!" Dr. Feinstein responded. "I'll be happy to help design the questionnaire. Just let me know when and where you want to meet and I'll be there."

As Lorraine placed the phone on the receiver, her eyes filled with tears. If she had been disillusioned by the reaction of some people to the news that she had gotten breast cancer, Dr. Feinstein redeemed her faith in humanity. His immediate and enthusiastic reaction energized her and gave her hope that this plan just might work!

With renewed vigor, she made her next call. It was to Mary Hibberd, the Suffolk County health commissioner and a medical doctor, who took Lorraine's call immediately, greeting her warmly and eager to hear what she had to say. At the time, Lorraine didn't know that Dr. Hibberd's mother had died of breast cancer.

As determined as she was to get her plan off the ground and as much as she believed in what she was doing, it was still intimidating for Lorraine to speak to the commissioner. She had seen the tall, slender brunette several times on television and was always struck by her openness and accessibility, but somehow talking to her "in person" made Lorraine nervous.

But before she could get the first word out, Dr. Hibberd put her at ease. "I saw your picture in *Newsday*," she said, "and it really looks like you shook them up at the CDC!"

The nervousness Lorraine felt dissipated into laughter and she once again described her plan, aware that she was venturing into unknown territory by asking an appointed official to collaborate with her on a major science project. She girded herself for a polite turndown.

But Dr. Hibberd was one of many people in Suffolk County – both professional and nonprofessional – who had agonized about the rising rate of breast cancer in the region and who was especially disturbed that the disease's mortality rate in Suffolk was among the highest in the state.

She asked Lorraine several questions about the design of the questionnaire, where the funding would come from, and which other people would be participating in the project. Lorraine didn't have all the answers, but she promised to get back to Dr. Hibberd as soon as she did. And then, as if handing her a gift, Dr. Hibberd agreed to meet with Lorraine to discuss the plan further.

The following week, only three weeks from the day that she'd envisioned her plan and jotted down its outline in her kitchen, Lorraine found herself sitting at a gigantic mahogany conference table at the Suffolk County Board of Health with Dr. Feinstein, Dr. Hibberd, Dr. Mahfouz H. Zaki, Suffolk County's assistant commissioner of health, and Michael LoGrande.

"Is this really happening?" she asked herself incredulously. The question was unnecessary, since the ensuing conversation made it clear that everyone present was eager to contribute in any possible way to a greater understanding of the scourge that was afflicting and killing so many women in Suffolk County. When a couple of hours had gone by and everyone stood up to shake hands and say goodbye, Lorraine's plan was on its way to being implemented.

Drs. Feinstein, Hibberd, and Zaki agreed to design a questionnaire that asked West Islip residents their health histories, where they lived, how long they had lived in the county, what kind of work they did, what their sources of drinking water were, and if any of them had breast cancer, benign breast disease, or no cancer at all. In short, a questionnaire that couldn't be challenged as "unscientific" or its results dismissed as "anecdotal."

Lorraine was exhilarated and eager to tackle the assignment the doctors had given her: to find funding for printing and distributing the questionnaire. One of them suggested she contact her Congressman, Tom Downey, which she and her friend Pat Nichols promptly did. Downey suggested they go to AC Type, an area printer, for a price quotation. The owner of the firm, Angie Carpenter (who would eventually be elected to the Suffolk County legislature) gave them a more-than-reasonable price and, excited by the project, called her old friend Ted Shiebler, Director of Public Relations at Good Samaritan Hospital, setting up an appointment on the spot. Lorraine and Pat went straight from Angie's office to Shiebler's office in Good Sam.

Shiebler's reputation for being accessible and going out of his way to help those in need was well deserved. "Ask Ted" was the usual response when anyone had a question, a worry, or a problem. True to his good name, he greeted Lorraine and her friend Pat Nichols with his hallmark courtesy and an attentive ear. With her words tumbling out, she told him of the willingness of Drs. Feinstein, Hibberd, and Zaki to help develop the questionnaire and then broached the subject at hand: Good Samaritan's endorsement of the project and funding.

Shiebler listened and nodded, giving an immediate and resounding yes to her first request. Like other regional hospitals, the doctors at Good Sam were operating on and treating more and more women with breast cancer, and they, too, were mystified by the escalating incidence of the disease. Unbeknownst to Lorraine, however, Shiebler's positive response was also based on the desire to remove the taint of a horrific scandal that had gravely damaged the good name of the institution five years before.

At that time, Richard Angelo, a registered nurse on the staff, was found to have engaged in a months-long pattern of injecting potentially deadly muscle relaxants, Pavulon and Anectine, into the intravenous lines of patients, watching them gasp desperately for breath and then "saving" their lives at the last minute – except that four patients died and as many as 10 may have died.

When the drugs were found in the apartment of the former Eagle Scout and volunteer fireman, Angelo – who was dubbed "Angel of Death" by the media – was arrested and immediately confessed to murder. A jury found him responsible for two counts of second-degree murder, one count of manslaughter, and one count of criminally negligent homicide, and he received the maximum sentence allowed by law, a prison term of 61 years to life.

Lorraine was delighted with Good Sam's endorsement and only slightly disappointed when Shiebler told her he'd get back to her about the financing, but with his fax machine buzzing, the phones ringing off the hook, and people flinging memos on the P.R. director's desk, she didn't want to take up any more of his time. As she got up to thank him and say goodbye, he stopped her cold.

"You're not going anywhere," he said good-naturedly. "This idea of yours is timely and important, and I think I can help it along in another way. Let's give it a try."

"Oh my God," Lorraine responded. "How did you know there were other problems? To be honest, I have no idea how to get the word out!"

Shiebler smiled and picked up the phone. "That's my business," he said.

Lorraine sat motionless as she heard Ted describe her idea, word for word, to the person on the other end of the phone. Every now and then he'd pause, listen, answer a question, and then do some more explaining. Finally, he handed Lorraine the phone. "Somebody wants to speak to you," he said.

"Hello," Lorraine said tentatively.

The somebody on the other end of the phone was Lou Grasso, managing editor of *Suffolk Life*, the county's main regional newspaper chain, who asked her to tell him about the mapping project in her own words. Without coming up for air, she repeated everything she had told Ted Shiebler, finally blurting out that she didn't know how she was going to get the survey to everyone in West Islip.

For a long minute there was no sound on the other end of the phone. At first Lorraine thought they had been disconnected.

"Hello, hello, are you there?" she said.

"Oh, I'm still here," Grasso responded. "Sorry about the silence, but I was just thinking how wonderful it is that there are still people like you in the world, people who aren't afraid to ask the hard questions and will do just about anything – within reason – to get answers. This sounds very reasonable to me."

Just a few weeks before, one of Grasso's proofreaders had been diagnosed with breast cancer, which had given him an up close and personal look at the nightmare of the diagnosis and the panic it creates. But his interest went even deeper. About 10 years earlier, he had learned of another "cluster" of health problems in the Suffolk County village of Bellport. Intrigued and disturbed by the many cases of leukemia, neurological problems, and birth defects in certain areas of the town, he had conducted his own informal survey, trudging from door to door to interview residents and ask them their theories.

He had learned that they all lived near a former nuclear facility where drums full of radioactive material were buried. Numerous "spills" had been reported over the years, which the residents considered an ominous sign since the site was situated near a well from which they got their drinking water.

Using the power of the press and a copy of a map that he had developed, Lou had called upon the state health department to clean up the site. Only a few weeks later, he watched as men in moon suits hauled away truckloads of contaminated waste, and, two years later, it didn't escape his attention that the "expert" who told him he had been cleaning up these "safe" sites for years died of cancer.

As fate would have it, Lou was sitting with *Suffolk Life*'s publisher, David Wilmott, a rangy six-footer who, at 51, still had an abundance of Huck Finn red hair. He and Lou shared a love for retrievers (Lou had goldens, Dave Labradors) as well as ocean fishing, and Dave often hosted their fishing trips on his 48-foot Ocean Super Sport boat.

Wilmott's ready smile, however, betrayed a ferocity of purpose. Blazing with journalistic zeal, he had begun his publishing career in 1961 with a solitary community newspaper in Riverhead that boasted a circulation of 9,000. By the early 1990s, he had expanded his empire to 35 newspapers with a collective circulation of over 500,000, adding a special *Summer Life* edition for the hordes of visitors who frequented the Island's East End from June to September.

In the maelstrom of hardball electoral races and subterranean goings-on that characterized Long Island's political scene, Wilmott routinely featured provocative interviews with opposing political candidates that served as often to illuminate their positions as to expose their inconsistencies. But he gained national renown – and not a few enemies – when, in 1967, he started publishing his objections to the Shoreham Nuclear Power Plant, insisting "in print" that the poorly designed structure be shut down.

For over 20 years, a relentless stream of editorials and articles appeared in the *Suffolk Life* chain of papers citing scientific evidence that the plant's low-level releases of radiation were dispersed over a ten-mile area and warning residents of the potential for a major meltdown that would result in radiation saturating Long Island and reaching as far as Boston and Washington, D.C., as well as an economic loss to Long Island that would amount to trillions of dollars.

In 1987, the plant was finally closed. A few years later, Wilmott was proud to be profiled in the annual edition of the book *Newsmakers* as "the man who killed nuclear energy in the United States."

True to his conviction that it was the duty of the press to investigate and open to public scrutiny issues that concerned his readership, it took Wilmott about one minute to give the nod to publishing Lorraine's survey.

"I'll tell you what the publisher and I have just decided," Lou said to Lorraine, who was still hanging on the phone with eager anticipation. "We've decided to publish that survey of yours on the front page – for the entire 11795 zip code of West Islip – so that every person in your town will see it. As for the price – it's on *Suffolk Life*!"

Lorraine was speechless. Fighting back tears, she struggled to find the words to thank Ted Shiebler and Lou Grasso and Dave Wilmott – all of them the antithesis of Elmer Gantry, she thought – three men she had never met before that day, who had opened up their hearts and generosity to her and her project.

Driving home, Lorraine pinched herself to make sure she wasn't dreaming. She actually took one hand off the wheel and pinched her face, then her thigh, then her arm. She didn't know quite what to do with all the good news she had just received. What she wanted to do was open her car window and shout it out to anyone and everyone she saw: "Hey, everyone, the answers are coming!" But she controlled the extravagant impulse and recited the words to herself.

By the time she pulled into her driveway, the reality of everything that had transpired that day sank in. She needed help designing a survey and had managed to find the right people. She needed help in getting the word out and, in this case too, had convinced some influential people to lend her assistance. As she sat in her car reviewing her weeks of nonstop lobbying and digesting the astounding results, she was struck by another reality: "I'm going to need lots more help!" And she set out to find it.

Chapter Four

Kitchen Revolutionaries

On August 5, 1992, just five months after Lorraine had breast cancer surgery, the brainchild she had dreamt up in her kitchen to chart the breast cancer incidence in her entire community became a reality. True to the promises she'd received, the entire questionnaire was published on the front page of *Suffolk Life*'s West Islip edition.

It had been formulated in a matter of weeks by some of the most prominent doctors and busiest health department officials in the county, embraced and spurred forward by the powers-that-be at a leading hospital, and published by a publisher and journalist who had established a precedent by featuring a health survey on the cover of a community newspaper.

All of them had pondered the high incidence of breast cancer in the region and agonized privately about the great number of their friends and family members who had been stricken with the disease. Many of them spoke about breast cancer as a "time bomb," viewing it as a deadly explosive that lay dormant in the bodies of innocent women until some mysterious trigger set it into action.

But what was the trigger – or triggers? When Lorraine suggested that at least one trigger may be something as simple as drinking water, the idea seemed to inflame their imaginations. Although the idea wasn't unfamiliar to them, they clearly thought that investigating the possible breast cancer–drinking water link was an idea whose time had come, a promising idea, a daring and bold idea. And such a simple idea – to ask the people of *one* community about their health histories, their sources of drinking water, and their incidence of breast cancer.

The survey did not ask questions about the flow of water; no one except the officials with access to maps of underground pipes really knows in which direction the water on a particular street flows. Rather, the survey was looking to answer a very specific question: Were there *clusters* of breast cancer in West Islip?

Lorraine suspected there were. But the scientists she had spoken with didn't seem to believe in clusters. To a person, they had told her that it was a "coincidence" that 20 women in an eight-block radius of her home had breast cancer. It was not the first time that her notion of clusters or hot spots would be dismissed by scientists for what they regarded as good reasons.

Apparent logic drives lay people to conclude that if a lot of people in one area have cancer, particularly a certain type of cancer, all they have to do is identify the cancer-causing agent to which those with the disease have been exposed and, theoretically at least, eliminate the toxic agent in order to prevent future cases of cancer.

So prevalent was this line of thinking that in 1989 alone, according to a survey by Daniel Wartenburg of the Robert Wood Johnson

Medical School in New Jersey, state health departments in the U.S. had received about 1,500 requests for cancer cluster investigations. But health officials were – and still are – unconvinced by the cluster theory, a fact that inspired the CDC, in 1990, to abandon routine investigations of cancer clusters.

The CDC and other health officials say that local groups often include different types of cancer that may not be triggered by the same carcinogen and that the people they survey were often diagnosed with cancer before they moved into the neighborhood in question. In addition, cancer has a long latency period, and its onset may be the result of genetic vulnerability or exposure to one or more carcinogens decades before that a person either may not have known about or may have forgotten. In short, researchers are unlikely to investigate a cancer cluster unless it is so consistently high that it is unlikely to be the result of pure chance.

Nevertheless, in a 2002 report, culminating yearlong research into the methods used by health agencies to investigate cancer clusters, reporters at *Newsday* concluded that investigative methods themselves might be flawed. They concluded that:

- The "chaotic system [is] designed more to mollify people… and the politicians who represent them than to reach scientifically valid conclusions about local cancer rates."

- While Long Island is widely regarded as the place where public concern about clusters is at its highest, the agency that does almost all local cluster investigations, the state health department, still uses methods that are assailed by activists, dismissed as ineffective by many scientists, and shunned by some states and the federal government.

- Investigations in New York are generally so superficial that they may be missing scientifically legitimate clusters. State officials say they have found solid evidence of clustering just three times out of the almost 350 investigations of alleged community clusters they've conducted since 1981.

- Evidence exists from sources – including the department's own cancer maps and the details of the reports it issues after each investigation – that cancer cases do indeed cluster in specific places and that New York's relatively cursory methods may be failing to detect some of those clusters.

All that said, over the years a number of carcinogens have been associated with human illness, such as vinyl chloride's link to angiosarcoma, diethylstilbestrol's (DES) link to gynecologic cancers in daughters of women who took the drug during pregnancy, and mesothelioma's link to asbestos.

In addition, Lorraine thought that the attitudes of the scientists were cavalier, and she found most of them oddly incurious. She knew of nine breast cancer cases on one block in a Nassau County community and, every day it seemed, heard of new clusters that people suspected – but couldn't prove – were the result of electromagnetic fields from power lines or waste products from materials like tungsten, celluloid, asbestos, and adhesives that spewed, unregulated, from factories in the region.

Increasingly, residents of Merrick, Bellmore, Wantagh, Hewlett, Woodmere, East Rockaway, Valley Stream, Oceanside, Port Washington, Great Neck, Roslyn, and Massapequa were reporting clusters of cancer to county and state health departments.

In Farmingdale, Suffolk County, the principal of Northside Elementary School said that 17 out of 42 employees had breast cancer, most of them having worked in the school for 20 years, and that school employees on the town's north side had high cancer rates that they suspected were caused by emissions of diesel fuel and toxic chemicals – such as Roundup, Arsenal, and WeatherBlok – that were used by the Long Island Rail Road to defoliate the area and rid it of rodents.

The principal had her own theories. In 1985, lightning struck the Wagner Brothers Seed Corporation in Farmingdale, which was three blocks from Northside School. A huge fire ensued, and the water used to fight the fire spread the chemical pesticides and fertilizers in the company's warehouse throughout the neighborhood. Sandbags were placed over the sewer drains to prevent the pesticides from reaching the sewers, which caused the saturated mixture to back up on sidewalks and lawns. Homeowners were told to drain their pools.

When cleanup crews arrived wearing head-to-toe protective clothing, they removed 1,300 cubic yards of contaminated soil from holes dug six feet deep in the neighborhood. Seven months

96

after the cleanup, the federal Environmental Protection Agency found that the contaminated soil had been improperly dumped in a Long Island Rail Road parking lot adjacent to the warehouse.

The Wagner brothers insisted that the entire incident was an act of God, and the Environmental Protection Agency said the problem was not their responsibility. Numerous people became sick after the fire, some debilitated and unable to work. For most residents, the region's high incidence of cancer was no mystery.

In other neighborhoods, high cancer rates were attributed to incinerators or dumpsites or to proximity to golf courses on which huge quantities of pesticides were used regularly.

In 1991, New York State Attorney General Robert Abrams released a study, "Toxic Fairways: Risking Groundwater Contamination from Pesticides on Long Island Golf Courses." The study looked at 107 courses in a 1,400-acre region and found that six pesticides, totaling nearly 10,000 pounds, were classified by the EPA as possible or probable human carcinogens. The report said that 200,000 pounds of dry bulk chemicals and close to 9,000 gallons of bulk liquid chemicals were used in one year alone on the golf courses of Long Island. Two of the chemicals, Dachthal and chlorothalonil, were detected in Long Island groundwater at the highest levels in the United States.

At the time, Lorraine did not know about all these cases, but she considered many of the scientists sneering at the concept of clusters to be Elmer Gantrys. When she received her issue of

Suffolk Life, however, and saw the survey on its front page, it was Christopher Columbus who came to mind.

"I knew that I was taking an uncharted course," she said, "but all I could think of was how many people once believed that the world was flat!"

Before she finished reading the survey, her phone began ringing off the hook.

Actually, it already had been ringing off the hook for the previous four weeks, after a lengthy article in the Long Island section of *The New York Times* detailed her efforts to enlist various experts to formulate a scientific grassroots survey of her community. Within hours of the article's publication, she had been called to appear on CNN, ABC-TV's *Eyewitness News*, and CBS-TV's *Eye on America*, and interviewed for a *USA Today* article – the first of dozens if not hundreds of interviews that would follow.

The idea of one woman *not* believing "the experts" and taking matters into her own hands clearly captured the imagination of media people. To be sure, it was not as if challenging the authorities was such an unprecedented act; all of them knew about people throughout history who had done the same. The difference in this particular challenge was that it involved a map – a concrete, visible object that would either show or not show that Lorraine's suspicions were valid. Moreover, this map, unlike the inscrutable maps that scientific organizations produce, would be available to them and presumably comprehensible, and they couldn't wait to get their hands on it.

They called Lorraine constantly with questions, but the other calls she was now receiving had a different flavor. The survey on the cover of *Suffolk Life* had tapped an anxiety in West Islip that had been festering for years. Finally, the callers told Lorraine, they had someone to whom they could express their fears and suspicions. Better yet, they could answer the survey's questions, which they did in astounding numbers.

Overnight, bags of completed questionnaires began to flood the mailbox of Good Samaritan Hospital, the address listed on the survey. The telephone numbers listed on the survey were those of Pat Nichols and John Pace Jr.'s real estate office. While Lorraine had been filled with optimism that people would respond to the survey, she was nonetheless astonished – and overwhelmed – by the response.

Each afternoon, her friend Pat Nicols would pick up the surveys from Good Sam and deliver them to Lorraine's home to be sorted. In addition, her son's secretary, Donna Ketcham, brought her copies of the telephone calls each evening. Within days, the surveys and phone messages began to pile up on her dining room table and chairs, her living room couch, her kitchen counter, her night table.

One evening, Donna delivered 25 telephone messages. But instead of being pleased that so many people had responded to the survey, Lorraine let out a deep groan. Sorting through the pile, she found herself talking out loud: "What do all these horrible cancer cases mean? Who will believe this? What am I supposed to do now?"

She had already spoken to several of her friends and neighbors, asking if they'd be willing to "sort out" the surveys when they arrived. But she hadn't anticipated the great quantity of surveys or the kind of help she'd need. What had begun as an exciting and even important project had become a nightmare.

Sipping her tea each morning, driving to various appointments during the day, lying in bed at night, all she could do was ruminate about what to do with all the information she was receiving in bundles each day. Beside herself, she called Lou Grasso.

Having worked in busy, deadline-driven newsrooms for years, Lou was accustomed to pressing demands and urgent requests. In his early 60s, the paunchy, gray-haired six-footer – who was often compared to The Daily Planet's editor, Perry White, in the Superman comic book series – seemed to have the ideal, unflappable temperament for such frenzied environments, the kind of disposition he so admired in his beloved golden retrievers and that was perfectly suited to the long hours he spent on weekends angling for weakfish, flounder, fluke, and bluefish in the Peconic and Great South Bays of Long Island. Even as a fisherman, Lou knew how to tackle big problems, which he did one blistering summer day in 1982 when he reeled in a 94-pound white marlin – the largest on record from the Atlantic Ocean – ultimately mounting the big fish in the den of his home.

But the rumpled-looking editor with the crooked tie and rolled-up sleeves ran his office with militaristic discipline, firing orders and news updates to his staff from his glass-enclosed command post. Behind a desk piled high with papers (and a bowl full of dog biscuits), Lou – who was known as "Chief" in his newsroom – took Lorraine's call immediately, not at all expecting her opening salutation.

"Help!" she cried into the phone.

As it happened, "help" was another of Lou's specialties. Some years before, when a young boy wrote to him that his father needed dialysis, Lou published an article that raised $12,000. He had initiated a Christmas drive for poor children that yielded piles of toys and a good deal of money, worked tirelessly to raise awareness about protecting the environment of a Suffolk County state park, and contributed countless hours to the Rotary Club, the Chamber of Commerce, and a community hospital board.

But when he heard Lorraine's plaintive "Help," Lou immediately recalled a fund he had started called The Impossible Dream, in which children with disabilities were treated to trips to Disneyland. He knew that her project was perceived as an impossible dream, and the solution-oriented editor had the perfect solution.

To "make sense of the whole thing," he told Lorraine, she needed someone who would lend credibility to the survey, who had the credentials and experience to deflect or negate any criticism she might receive from institutions or science experts who would take any and every opportunity to discredit the survey's findings.

"But who?" Lorraine wailed into the phone.

Promising to call her back, Lou called Vicky Katz, a journalist he knew from her days as editor of *The Smithtown Messenger* and, more recently, as the director of public relations at Stony Brook University. Vicky was the ultimate resource person, and, sure enough, she suggested just the kind of person Lou was looking for: Roger Grimson.

The name rang a bell. While they had never met, Lou had followed a series of *Newsday* articles that described the study Dr. Grimson was conducting into the epidemiology of mysterious cases of cancer that had stricken nine Stony Brook University students a few years after they graduated.

The minute Lou made contact with Dr. Grimson, he recognized him as an approachable and accessible person who, indeed, was interested in the mapping project. He told Lou that he would do anything he could to help solve the Long Island breast cancer mystery.

When Lou called Lorraine back to tell her that Dr. Grimson had agreed to help analyze the survey's data, she was overcome with relief. The piles of paper that surrounded and all but drowned her could now, she believed, be handed over to a scientist able to make sense of it all. But when she expressed this notion to Lou, he summarily nixed the idea.

"Roger can analyze the data," he said. "But you have to get it together."

"What do you mean?" Lorraine inquired, completely befuddled by his directive.

"It's simple," he said. "*You* have to take the surveys and get them into some kind of order. Maybe get some friends to help you. You have to tell Roger the what and where and when of all this stuff, to chart it, to map it."

Lorraine told him that she already had begun sorting the surveys with a few friends, but that the mounting piles were "too much" for them to handle. "That's easy," he responded. "You need more woman power!"

His suggestion was so simple, so obvious, that Lorraine felt embarrassed – and also relieved. "Is that it?" she laughed. "I can do that!" She told Lou that she wanted to meet Dr. Grimson, and he promised to arrange a meeting. A couple of hours later, Dr. Grimson called her, and a few days later they met at her home, after which Lorraine had a better idea of how to map the surveys and a feeling of assurance that the analysis of her mapping project was in the best possible hands.

But as she set about soliciting more friends and neighbors to help her, she had no idea what a hornet's nest the survey had created for Lou and *Suffolk Life*.

Unlike Lorraine, Lou was receiving lots of negative feedback. "How could you publish *that thing* and risk panicking everyone on Long Island?" a state health department official blasted him. "I'm getting calls from hundreds of people – and they want answers," a local politician chided him. "What am I supposed to do, move my wife and children and work to another community?" a West Islip resident cried over the phone.

Lou and Dave Wilmott were as concerned as their critics about a widespread panic. To avert such an event, Lou published editorial upon editorial that reminded his readers that the cancer scare *might* be an isolated phenomenon and that urged them not to jump to any premature conclusions. Elizabeth Tonis, one of *Suffolk Life*'s ace reporters, wrote dozens of articles that followed the project's progress and gave human faces to the women who were mapping the results of the survey.

In addition, the paper succeeded in placing the project in a larger context by constantly challenging the state health department to update its obsolescent cancer registry, which was at least five years behind in collating data. Keypunch operators had been laid off because of budget cuts, and the record-keeping was so antiquated that clerks wrote the data on three-by-five cards that continued to pile up, unanalyzed, for months on end. In an age when industries, homes, businesses, and even state lotteries were increasingly driven by computers – the limousines of data collection – the state health department was mired in the horse-and-buggy era of papers and pencils and, as a result, drastically overdue reports.

Equally troubling was the fact that a lot of cancer deaths in the registry were reported as deaths due to respiratory distress or heart failure or other end-of-life symptoms, which effectively rendered the reportage of the state's breast cancer mortality rates inaccurate.

The newspaper also urged its readers to start working with local hospitals to insist, collectively, that the cancer registry be updated.

These problems were not on Lorraine's front burner, however. Right after speaking with Roger Grimson, she set about convincing, cajoling, persuading, and generally rounding up what would become her Kitchen Cabinet.

Pat Nicols, a friend who Lorraine considered her soul mate, was already on board and had begun to sort the surveys with Lorraine. Diagnosed with breast cancer eight years earlier, she had accompanied Lorraine to the second meeting with Dr. Hibberd at the Board of Health and had been her staunchest supporter from the time Lorraine was diagnosed through her radiation and chemotherapy treatments.

Lorraine had called upon Pat often in the preceding months, sometimes with specific questions, other times simply to cry. Although Pat juggled a full-time job as an R.N. at Good Samaritan with raising three kids and going to various social and professional functions with her husband, Joseph, an oral surgeon, she was the first to volunteer for the mapping project. Now Lorraine wanted

Pat's practical advice on how to go about following Lou Grasso's directive.

"I was thinking of asking some of the women I know with breast cancer to help me collate the surveys," Lorraine told Pat over the phone, "but I'm not sure if that's a good idea because so many of them are in the middle of chemo or suffering from depression or just trying to keep their heads above water."

"I think it's a great idea!" Pat responded. "They're looking for answers too – and 'doing something' about finding those answers will be empowering."

When she hung up the phone, Lorraine was charged with energy. She dialed her close friend Maria Diorio, who worked the 3-to-11 p.m. shift as a registrar in the emergency room of Good Sam. Though she had seen plenty of "bad stuff" in her 11 years there, she had never heard of the breast cancer "epidemic" on Long Island and had no relatives with the disease. But she had plenty of trouble in her own life.

A couple of years earlier, Maria's mother, Vincenza Melucci, had died, leaving Maria with an empty room in her home and a broken heart. Shortly after the death, Maria's husband, Ed, was diagnosed with chronic lymphatic leukemia, for which he was treated with chemotherapy and gamma globulin. In addition, Ed Jr., who was 30, had been diagnosed with an autoimmune disease and placed on steroids.

Young Eddie, who was forced to go on disability at the time, was married to a vibrant young woman named Pam Chapman Diorio, a fifth-grade teacher at the Udall Middle School in West Islip. They were the parents of a golden-haired, dark-eyed toddler named Samantha, and Pam was nine months pregnant with their second child when she learned that the baby boy had died in utero.

Maria was also involved with her other children, Anthony, who was 33 and in the Navy, and Donna Martinez, who at 32 worked part-time in the accounts payable department of Good Samaritan Hospital and was the mother of an energetic three-year-old boy, T.J., and baby Alyssa, both of whom provided their grandmother with hours of joy.

Although Maria had enough troubles to keep anyone preoccupied and depressed, she was an eternal optimist who never looked at the dark side of life and fervently believed that God gave problems only to those who could handle them. She instantly volunteered to help Lorraine with the mapping project.

Pam volunteered as well and often told people that seeing how valiantly the women with breast cancer coped with their adversity gave her strength to cope with her baby's death. She also convinced her sister-in-law Alexandra Chapman to join the project. Alex, a registered nurse with three school-age children, was in her early 30s and had been diagnosed with breast cancer a day after Lorraine's diagnosis. Alex and Pam gave unstintingly to the project, day after day, week after week, month after month.

From day one, Maria took charge, becoming the de facto "captain" of the Kitchen Revolutionaries, organizing meetings, setting up schedules, delegating jobs, coordinating the entire project. She clearly had the knack of juggling several priorities at one time, which anyone could see by simply observing her in action. This included the care of her granddaughter Alyssa, who accompanied Maria to every meeting.

"C'mon, girls, let's go!" she'd say when she found the volunteers sitting at the kitchen table eating bagels and sipping coffee. She handed some of the women three-by-five index cards on which to transcribe the data from the surveys, charged others with alphabetizing the streets and putting the street numbers in order, and instructed others to locate the addresses on the map of West Islip Lorraine had obtained from the Suffolk County Water Authority. Over the course of the 18 months that the project lasted, Maria – proving that if you want something done ask a busy person to do it – was the only one of the heroic volunteers to never, ever miss a day!

Donna Ketcham, a bubbly teenager with honey-blonde hair, went to work at Pace Real Estate Services in 1989 as John Pace Jr.'s secretary; three years later, when the survey was published, she was dating her boss. The survey listed the office's number, but no one expected the avalanche of calls that poured in. Donna, poised and articulate, handled the calls with a degree of compassion and expertise that belied her youth.

In fact, when she was a toddler, fate had all but robbed her of her youth. At the age of two, with her father out of town on business, Donna was with her mother when a man broke into their home, murdered her mother, and tried to drown Donna. Years of nightmares followed, but the only obvious "symptom" she displayed as she emerged into adulthood was a deep compassion for people who were going through hard times.

The calls never stopped. "Why was the survey done?" some callers asked Donna. "How should I answer question number 6?" (or 14 or 30?) others wanted to know. "When will we know the answers?" literally dozens of people asked. At the very least, there were 10 phone calls a day; some days there were 25.

Unfailingly polite and empathetic, Donna would speak to the callers, offer them comfort, write down their questions, place all the relevant things they said on a neat list, and drive to Lorraine's home each night to deliver the information. Lorraine, in turn, would call every person back, often getting off the phone after midnight, completely talked out and blurry with exhaustion.

Donna was never lost for words, fielding even the most difficult question or belligerent caller with patience and grace. But there were exceptions. Actually, there was only one exception. One day, she got a call from a woman who had seen Lorraine on Long Island's News 12 TV and wanted to know if the mapping project would include her own town of Massapequa.

"I'm so sorry," Donna responded, "but Massapequa isn't part of the survey. However, I'll have Lorraine call you because she's now lecturing around the Island and telling a lot of other communities how to set up their own mapping projects. Please give me your name."

The soft-spoken woman told her that her name was Carol Baldwin. "I'm just a regular housewife," she added, "but the name may ring a bell because my sons are actors. Did you ever hear of Alec Baldwin?" Donna shrieked and squealed. "Oh my God!" She listed half-a-dozen movies she had seen featuring the woman's famous son and promised that Lorraine would call her back that evening, which she did.

The women became fast friends and Carol became a frequent guest, sometimes staying overnight at Lorraine's home for weeks at a time, often with her granddaughter Jill. When Carol expressed interest in "getting more involved," Lorraine suggested that she start an organization to fund research. Lorraine persuaded her husband John to form the 501 (c) 3, pro bono of course, and recruited the original board members of what eventually became the Carol M. Baldwin Breast Cancer Research Fund, Inc. They included Carol herself; radiation oncologist Dr. Allen G. Meek; Dr. Michael Maffetone, Director and CEO of Stony Brook Hospital; Suffolk County activist Joan Therese Hudson and John Pace. The organization would go on to raise over $1 million and, years later, when Lorraine worked at Stony Brook, she was implemental in getting the university to name The Carol M. Baldwin Breast Care Center in her friend's honor.

Meanwhile, Donna stayed with the project – every day – for its entire existence, growing closer to Lorraine each time they met. They had a true affinity for one another – they even looked alike! Over the course of the survey, Donna became engaged to John Jr., and she and Lorraine grew closer than ever.

Since speaking with Pat Nicols and Maria Diorio two weeks previously, Lorraine had been glued to her phone, putting together what would become a close-knit group of women who were committed to "getting answers" to the disease they either feared or had.

She bumped into Fredricka O'Connor in the produce section of the local supermarket, Grand Union, and told her about the project. Fredi, a nurse at West Islip High School and the mother of four, had so many friends and neighbors with breast cancer that she immediately volunteered to help file and alphabetize the surveys. Over the course of the project, no matter how busy she was or what other pressing demands life made on her, she was indefatigable in working on the mapping project.

Mary McCauley also lived on a dead-end street in West Islip, near the water. In her early 30s, she had been diagnosed with breast cancer a few months earlier, but in spite of her arduous treatments she proved to be one of the project's best organizers, filing the results of the survey methodically so the data could never be challenged by skeptics or cynics.

Jackie Paserb, whose husband, John, had been Lorraine's high school music teacher, had lived a quarter-mile from the bay in West Islip for over 40 years. The mother of three and a school nurse at St. John the Baptist High School, Jackie had no family history of breast cancer but had been diagnosed with the disease at the same time Lorraine was.

When she bumped into Lorraine at a luncheon, they had an exchange that was becoming chillingly familiar to hundreds of Long Island women: "I have breast cancer," Lorraine said. "You're kidding – me too," Jackie responded, agreeing immediately to join the project and becoming invaluable in sorting the surveys into avenues, streets, lanes, roads, byways, and highways.

Pat Licata, a North Babylon resident and mother of two, didn't have breast cancer, but many of her friends and neighbors did. She worked tirelessly on the project and spent dozens of evenings speaking publicly at various functions and fund-raisers to inform the community what the project was all about and why, in fact, it was long overdue.

Virginia "Ginny" Regnante had been diagnosed eight years earlier. In her middle 50s, the mother of five was no longer working in real estate sales when she agreed to help. Outspoken and bubbling with both personality and questions, Ginny joined the group with zeal, visiting the offices of politicians with Lorraine to keep them up to date on the project and to let them know what *they* could do to further breast cancer awareness and improve legislation that affected women's health.

Jane Tinnelli, the sister-in-law of Lorraine's niece, was in her late 30s and the Kitchen Revolutionaries' fund-raising chairwoman for Good Samaritan Hospital's Breast Center, a division that had been established a few months after Lorraine's diagnosis in response to the frightening incidence of the disease in West Islip. Jane also lived on a dead-end street in West Islip and only a few months later, she, too, would be diagnosed with breast cancer. Jane's mother, Joan Ardito, also joined the project, immediately volunteering to sort the volumes of mail that continued to pour in.

These were the women who stayed with the project from beginning to end, balancing the busyness of their lives with the imperative they felt to find out why they or so many of their friends were being afflicted with breast cancer. But the project would never have proceeded with such dispatch if it hadn't been for other women who were also there at the beginning, volunteering their time in Lorraine's home to help get the project off the ground.

Among them was Kathy Annino, a nurse at Southside Hospital and a breast cancer survivor who lived on a dead-end street in the Great South Bay section of West Islip, and Cathleen Chapey, an elementary school teacher with seven children, who somehow found the time to help with sorting out the responses to what would become the project's direct mailing efforts.

Then there was Peggy Quinn, a friend of Lorraine's for 30 years and a former second-grade teacher, who lived with her husband, Pete, on another dead-end street in West Islip. They had raised six daughters, and Peggy said she would "do anything" to make sure that her kids and grandkids didn't suffer the ravages of a disease that "might" be avoided by changing the environment.

There was Rita Giorgini, whose husband was on the board of Good Samaritan Hospital and a physician on its staff, who stopped Lorraine in mid-sentence when asked to join the project. "Whatever I can do!" she exclaimed.

Mary Fezza was a West Babylon resident who felt strongly about Lorraine's mission and supported it unequivocally. A receptionist in a doctor's office in West Islip, Mary was diagnosed with breast cancer in her early 30s and, a few years later, would die of the disease. Her husband, Alex, who was on board from the beginning, continued to be involved in finding answers to the breast cancer scourge on Long Island as a board member of another activist group Lorraine established toward the end of the mapping project.

Evelyn Demers, a nurse, joined the project, but her hectic schedule didn't allow her to help with the nitty-gritty details. Married to a surgeon and with many domestic responsibilities and social events to attend, she remained a stalwart supporter of the mapping plan, speaking up at the increasing number of engagements to which members of the project were invited as "special guests."

Madeline Cerone – Lorraine's sister-in-law's sister-in-law – also lived on a dead-end street near the bay in West Islip. A housewife with two grown children, she had been diagnosed with breast cancer in the late 1980s.

On literally a do-or-die mission, Lorraine completed her ferocious campaign in less than three weeks. By the time Labor Day rolled around, women in groups of two and four and seven and ten were visiting her home every day, from ten in the morning to two in the afternoon, sifting through the hundreds of surveys that were pouring in.

Juggling family responsibilities and jobs – and, in the case of many of the women, radiation and chemotherapy treatments that made them tired, nauseated, and depressed – they managed to carve out an hour or two here, three or four hours there, to volunteer their time in the first-ever epidemiological study to be initiated by a breast cancer patient.

In many ways that was the easy part. For many of the women, less easy was being assailed by media people who had all but camped in Lorraine's driveway and in front of her home and the neighboring homes and driveways of her brothers-in-law. As they walked the gauntlet from their cars to the front door, the women found themselves fielding questions that ranged from the personal to the political.

"Do you have breast cancer?" one reporter would yell, as another shouted, "Why are you doing this?" TV reporters, many emerging from trucks topped with satellite dishes and surrounded by camera crews, asked opinions about the latest health department bulletin or the goal of the survey. "Is the problem worse in your community than in others?" one particularly insistent reporter asked day after day. Yet another, citing data from the state's outdated and inaccurate cancer registry, asked, "Why are more women dying of the disease in Suffolk County than in Nassau County?"

Radio reporters, toting tape recorders and microphones and eager to preempt their TV and print colleagues with a "scoop," elbowed their way to the walkway to fire their questions: "Aren't you causing a panic?" "Do you think your drinking water is contaminated?" "Do you really believe in cancer clusters?"

Most of the women had no experience with the media and some were frankly terrified, covering their faces as they emerged from their cars and running down Lorraine's walk through her front door. In addition to feeling inadequate about answering the questions that were fired at them every day, they struggled with the age-old question that confronts every patient with a serious illness – to tell or not to tell – to "go public" or not.

The majority of the volunteers were employed outside their homes and faced the prejudice that cancer patients experienced routinely in the early 1990s in their workplaces: the looks, the avoidance, and, most intimidating, the threat that they'd be let go under a pretense that had nothing to do with job performance.

Even scarier to them was the possibility that their treatments would fail, necessitating a bone marrow transplant. Ironically, this dreaded possibility served to dissipate some of the fear they had in speaking to reporters.

Kitchen Revolutionaries

It hadn't escaped the attention of the Kitchen Revolutionaries that more and more Long Island women needed the transplants but were denied them by insurance companies claiming they were "experimental" – and that those women *had* gone public in hiring lawyers and calling upon the formidable support of Republican Senator Alfonse D'Amato to fight the insurance companies, invariably winning their cases when the outrageousness of the insurance companies' decisions became known.

These battles, as well as an increasingly positive public response to the project, ultimately broke down the barrier between the desire of the volunteers to guard their privacy and the compelling need to come out of the closet of secrecy. To be sure, they were inspired by Lorraine's example. She had already been featured in *Working Woman* magazine and appeared on ABC-TV's *Eyewitness News* with N.J. Burkett in the first of what would become an award-winning series of shows. In addition, she had appeared on CBS-TV's *Eye on America* with Dan Rather, CNN's *Earth Matters*, *The Maury Povich Show* and other national and international broadcasts, including those that aired in Canada and Australia. And the mapping project was always in the public eye through an ongoing series of articles by Liz Tonis in *Suffolk Life*.

Through Lorraine's example and the constant encouragement of Maria Diorio, the volunteers began to speak up. John Pace, a gracious host and enthusiastic supporter of the project, served literally as an "in house" counsel when legal questions arose, often advising the women about the narrow but accurate ways in which they could describe both themselves and their work.

Because none of them were scientists or doctors, he said, and no conclusions from the survey had yet been reached, they couldn't say much more than that they "suspected" they lived in a breast cancer cluster and they "hoped to find some answers." The volunteers' lack of experience with the media turned out to be to their advantage, since many of their answers came forth with blunt, unrehearsed honesty.

"I'm here because I and a whole lot of my neighbors have breast cancer and we don't know why," one Kitchen Revolutionary stated. "I never read the latest health department report," said another, "but whatever it said doesn't mean anything to me when I'm going for chemotherapy." From yet another woman: "I don't need a bulletin to know that too many women here and all over the country are dying from breast cancer." And "Panic? If 20 or 25 women within a few blocks – lots of them in their 30s and 40s – have breast cancer, that's a pretty good reason to panic, don't you think?"

All at once, women who had led productive but unpublicized lives saw their words quoted in local and regional newspapers, heard themselves on the radio and watched their images on TV. Neighbors stopped them in the streets with words of congratulation and support. Local shopkeepers greeted them like Hollywood celebrities. Letters of admiration from long-lost friends arrived at their doors. All this served to deepen their conviction about the rightness of their mission and to keep them focused.

And focus they did. On a map of West Islip that was so large – 10 feet long – it had to be moved from the kitchen table to the dining room table, they placed the surveys in categories: breast cancer, benign breast disease, and no breast disease. Every day, more surveys poured in and by early October, the women were astonished to realize that they numbered over 1,000!

The original plan had been to pinpoint the data by using the little colored pins that traditionally dot epidemiological maps. That idea was promptly abandoned when the women realized that the pins could easily fall off the map and get lost and they would never be able to carry the map to TV stations or public functions to show it off. They opted, instead, for magic markers: bright yellow to denote breast cancer, pink for benign breast disease, and blue for no breast cancer.

Painstakingly, some of the women proceeded to mark the map block by block, lane by lane, avenue by avenue, street by street, while others alphabetized and filed the surveys, and still others visited homes in the community to help residents complete the surveys. The long and cumbersome lists they worked from contained adhesive address labels that were earmarked to be sent to residents who hadn't responded to the initial mailing. They were so long and cumbersome, in fact, that they were finally placed on the floor, stretching from the dining room to the bedroom of Lorraine's spacious home. Before long, the hardy volunteers were suffering from backaches and eyestrain!

"It's ridiculous!" Lorraine exclaimed to Ted Scheibler when she called to update him on the project's progress. "Most of us have breast cancer, and now we're getting back problems and eye problems!" She had told the right person. Ted suggested that the women simply resend the surveys to all the addresses since those who had already filled them out would simply discard them. While most of the women knew that there were "several thousand" residents of West Islip, the list reminded them that the "small" area in which they lived included nearly 9,000 households – 8,940, to be exact.

As they plotted the map they talked about everything, on the lighter side their kids, dinner menus, a sale, or the latest gossip. On the heavier side, they discussed their cancer treatments and shared their fears. But a day never passed that they were not forced to deal with two unpleasant realities. One was the increasing number of complaints from Lorraine's neighbors about the constant traffic, parked cars, and TV trucks in front of their homes. Moving the project, however, was not an option, since the group had no money and quitting in midstream was completely out of the question. The second concern was finding the money to mail the survey to the residents of West Islip who hadn't responded to the one published in *Suffolk Life*.

They needn't have worried. From the day the *Times* article appeared in August, it was clear to John Pace that his wife's idea was "something big" and that the volunteers eventually would need formal status and lots of money to proceed with their plan. Working nights and weekends to assure that the group was formalized to the letter of the law, he contributed his legal expertise pro bono to apply for a Certificate of Incorporation and, a few months later, for nonprofit status (a 501(c)(3) organization).

In addition, he called his old friend, Republican State Senator Owen Johnson, to set up a meeting between the senator and Lorraine. No one could plead her case better, John knew, not even a lawyer such as himself. And plead her case she did, telling the senator that the Kitchen Revolutionaries needed funding to be able to afford a mailing. It didn't take much convincing.

Like other politicians on Long Island, Johnson was keenly aware of the breast cancer problem and the lack of progress that had been made in explaining it. He told Lorraine that she needed a grant and he'd try to get it. A few days later, the application papers arrived at her home, and John filled them out and mailed them back. Lorraine was elated, imagining that within weeks she'd have funds for the mailing and, hopefully, enough money to find an office and set up shop *outside* her home. She was unprepared for how sluggishly the wheels of government bureaucracy turned.

The following Monday, she once again called Democratic Congressman Thomas Downey, who had been so helpful to her in suggesting a company for printing and distributing the WIBCC's questionnaire. The dashing representative had gained notoriety for being the youngest person ever elected to Congress and although Lorraine's husband was unhappy that his wife was enlisting the support of a Democrat, Lorraine didn't care. The issue at hand was more important than any political party!

Downey took Lorraine's call immediately and asked her if she had investigated the printing costs as he had suggested. In fact, she had, not only visiting AC Type but spending weeks visiting over a dozen printers in Nassau and Suffolk and Queens, fastidiously making a list of their price quotations, packaging deals, and delivery times before accepting the firm he had originally recommended.

She had also gotten back to Ted Shiebler at Good Samaritan to tell him how grateful she was that he had lent the survey project the prestigious name of the hospital, thus giving it an important "Good Housekeeping Seal of Approval." But that was not the only thing on her mind. Bustling into the hospital toting sheaves of price quotations in a manila folder, she asked again if the institution would be willing to pay for any or all of the survey's printing and distribution costs.

Shiebler told her she might have to obtain a grant for the printing and mailing costs and that he would let her know about her request for the office space.

As she spoke with him, Lorraine felt deflated. She had amassed a good deal of information and enjoyed a productive conversation with both Congressman Downey and Ted Shiebler, but it all seemed to add up to another dead end. As she left Shiebler's office, she realized she was no nearer to getting the survey mailed than she had been at the beginning of her quest, and no nearer to finding office space for the project.

And the firestorm of criticism from her brothers-in-law still had not abated. In fact, their complaints about the unrelenting stream of media people whose cars and trucks blocked their driveways, disrupted the peace of the neighborhood, and infringed on their privacy grew louder. The pressure was immense. John worked closely with his brothers in real estate, politics, and legal ventures and, with his brother Anthony, shared a law practice, Pace & Pace, which was one of the most powerful in Suffolk County. Tension between them about the mapping project was growing daily.

The imperative to Lorraine was obvious: change the status quo *immediately* or risk a family feud of pervasive, long-standing, irreparable damage. The status quo, of course, was the mapping project all the women considered their "baby," which none of them would ever contemplate abandoning. The only solution to the "neighbor problem" and the chorus of daily complaints seemed to be the grant money that the Kitchen Revolutionaries hoped would be forthcoming from Senator Johnson's office.

Lorraine recognized that a mailing would reach everyone who hadn't responded to the survey, but when she did the math she felt – for the first time since the mapping project began – that the whole project might come to a crashing, dead-end halt. She figured that 1,000 stamps – even using bulk rate – came to over $2,000. And printing 7,000 surveys had to be at least a couple thousand more. She needed roughly $5,000, but the group's net worth was zero.

Up to this point every member had paid her own expenses, and Lorraine had more than dipped into the rent money she received from the house her father had left her for all the meals, telephone bills, and travel costs. When she computed the cost of a mailing, it was so outrageous that she burst out laughing! Breast cancer had transformed her into a fearless crusader, a woman who considered everything but death negotiable.

Problems were made for solutions, she thought to herself as she pondered exactly what to do and who else to call for help. She was afraid that data collected from only 1,000 West Islip residents would be dismissed out of hand by experts who were sure to say that the sample group was "too small" or that any conclusions professing a cancer cluster or that linked breast cancer and the environment were nothing less than "inconclusive."

Although Lorraine had become adept at asking questions, she knew that she now had to come up with some answers. As she lay tossing and turning in her bed at night, she thought of holding a fund-raiser but knew from experience that such an event required a tremendous amount of start-up money, organization, and time, as well as finding a venue, issuing invitations, mobilizing volunteers ... the list went on. Besides, it was unlikely that the Kitchen Revolutionaries could raise from their first event the kind of money that was needed.

She thought of placing flyers in every supermarket, library, storefront, and doctor's office in West Islip, petitioning the public to support the mailing in the same way they had supported the questionnaire. But that would cost more money and more time – neither of which they had.

She thought of joining other cancer advocacy groups on Long Island in *their* fund-raising efforts, but she knew how competitive each group was and how jealously they guarded their own agendas – and their own funds. By five a.m. every idea had hit a dead end. Finally, her mind cloudy with fatigue, she fell into a fitful sleep.

The next day was Saturday – no Kitchen Revolutionaries! Lorraine rose late. Padding around the kitchen in her nightgown and slippers, she poured her morning tea and gazed blankly out the window. After living in her home for so many years, she had grown so accustomed to the sight that she often took it for granted.

But this time her blank gaze turned to feelings of awe and appreciation as she beheld the panoramic sweep of the Great South Bay and, beyond it, the Robert Moses Causeway that led to the beach. She noticed with renewed wonder the sun reflecting off the water, boats large and small on their way to Fire Island, seagulls flying lazily overheard, an adorable family of ducks making its way across the water, and the last swan she'd see till spring gliding over the water like a graceful ballerina.

It hadn't escaped her notice, however, that the dozens of clam boats that once filled the bay from early morning to late evening had vanished. So numerous were they just a few years before that clammers would jump from boat to boat comparing their catches. Now the boats and the fishermen were gone. She thought there might be a connection between the decrease in the Great South Bay's shellfish population and an increase in breast cancer incidence, and suspected that an electroplating company that had closed its doors in 1985, might be responsible. Just a few days earlier she had learned that the company, which was two miles from her home, had been dumping cadmium, chromium, and cyanide in the waters since 1932. Months earlier, in fact, she had found a container of cadmium-based fungicide in her garage that had been used to treat her lawn and had wondered how many other homeowners treated their lawns with similar fungicides.

She knew that cyanide was poison, pure and simple, and had learned that cadmium, a heavy metal toxic to human health, could be inhaled or ingested in contaminated food and water, and was linked to bone demineralization and an increased risk of fractures, which was already a risk for post-menopausal women like her and many of her friends. "Cancer, too," she thought.

Emotion overcame her as she pondered the irony of her situation. "Here I am in the most beautiful setting on God's earth," she thought to herself, "and it may be the very setting that's causing all this cancer."

The thought jolted her from appreciation to anger. Two days later she called Congressman Downey again, not only to update him on her meeting at Good Sam and tell him about her application for a grant from Senator Johnson, but also to reinforce to him the kitchen brigade's desperate need for money for a mailing. She learned that he had been doing some work of his own.

"I've got some good news," he told her. "I've just secured a $5,000 grant from Revlon for the printing and distribution costs of the survey!"

Lorraine was stunned. To think that a busy politician who spent most of his time in Washington had considered her request so important that he had placed it on the front burner of his priorities was simply staggering to her. She thanked the congressman profusely, but he would have none of it. "I live on Long Island with my wife and children," he said. "If I'm not interested in our cancer rates, then who should be?"

In less than a week – thanks to the Revlon grant – a gigantic mailing to the entire West Islip community went out from Good Samaritan Hospital, using the hospital's special bulk rate. The Kitchen Revolutionaries had folded and placed each survey in a number 10 envelope, with Lorraine, John and their daughter Lisa working into the wee hours of the morning – after everyone else had gone home – to get each pile of envelopes to the hospital for mailing. The women expected another avalanche of responses (which in fact they received), but their efforts didn't stop there.

They also were walking singly and in pairs through every neighborhood of their town, going from door to door asking women who hadn't filled in the survey to do so. And every day they continued to show up at Lorraine's house, on occasion toting assorted pastries, rolls, and bagels.

Every now and then, Lorraine greeted them in passing, running out the door on her way to an interview to get the word out that yes, she "suspected" there was a cancer cluster in her community, and no, she didn't believe the science experts were correct in dismissing such a phenomenon.

It didn't take long for her TV and newsprint interviews to strike a deep chord in people throughout the country. Every day she found dozens of letters in her mailbox, personal letters from Oregon to Ohio, Maine to Montana, New York to New Mexico – in short, from just about every state in the union. They were encouraging letters, tear-stained letters, angry letters. No one who wrote, however, was skeptical.

Not a single person who sat down to put his or her feelings and beliefs into print doubted that Lorraine and her crew would find what they were looking for: *proof* that cancer clusters existed and, just as important, that they were linked to "something" in the environment.

While she was heartened, and also anguished, by the letters, Lorraine knew that answering them was impossible, at least then. There was simply too much work to do and too many unforeseen circumstances to deal with. It didn't matter to her, or to any of the women, that the Kitchen Revolutionaries were sometimes perceived as a gaggle of smartly dressed women meeting in a luxurious waterfront home over coffee, assembling survey data as they looked out on a scene as beautiful as the French Riviera.

In truth, the women wore jeans, sweat suits, and nurses' uniforms as often as skirts and dresses, and the glamorous setting had done nothing to protect many of them against cancer.

Each day brought something new, and the beginning of November turned out to be an important milestone. Although John Pace had formed a not-for-profit organization called the Breast Cancer Coalition of Long Island the previous month, he had amended the name to reflect the location where the increasingly famous mapping project was actually taking place. On November 4, 1992, the group was reborn as the West Islip Breast Cancer Coalition, or the WIBCC.

Meanwhile, the women were too busy to realize that they were in the process of making history, and they certainly didn't anticipate how far-reaching and influential their mapping project would become – or the problems that would arise as their prominence grew.

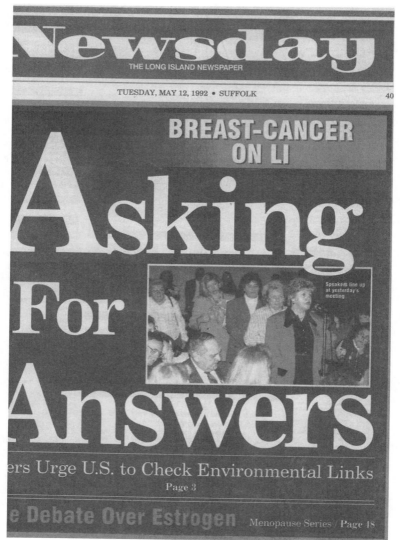

Lorraine Pace on the cover of Newsday, May 1992

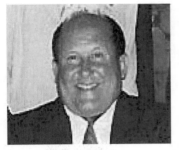

John Pace

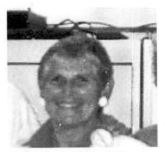

Barbara Balaban

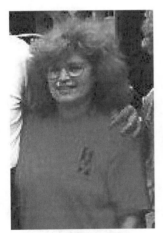

**Geri Barish
Long Island Breast
Cancer Coalition**

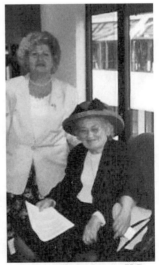

Lorraine Pace, former U.S.
Congresswoman Bella Abzug

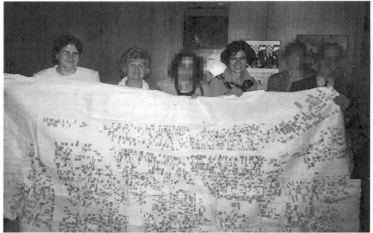

Holding map at the Smithsonian Institute in Washington, D.C., from left: Ruth Allen, head of the Environmental Protection Agency; Lorraine Pace, Dr. Devra Lee Davis

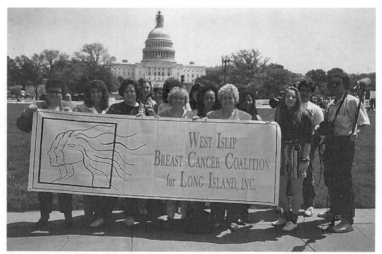

Members of the West Islip Breast Cancer Coalition lobbying in Washington D.C. in 1993.

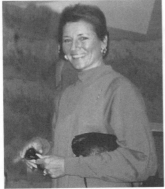

Diane Sackett Nannery

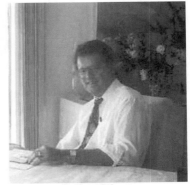

Dr. Roger Grimson

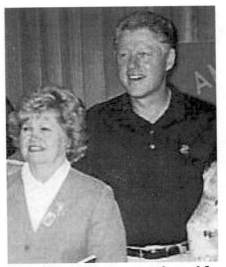

**President Clinton meeting with
Lorraine Pace in Suffolk
County on Long Island**

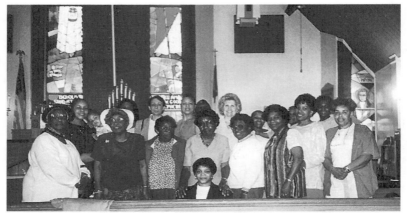

Lorraine Pace speaking at the Bethel AME church in Copiague in 1994 to raise awareness of breast cancer issues. The meeting resulted in the formation of Long Island's first minority breast cancer group, Sisters for Sisters (now called Sisters Network).

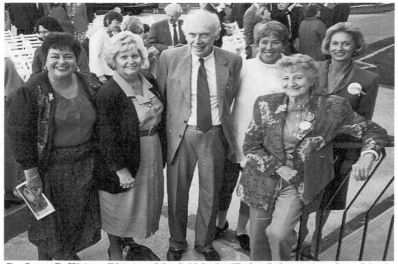

Dr. James D. Watson, Director of the Cold Spring Harbor Laboratory on Long Island, meeting with activists, from left: Ginny Regnante, Lorraine Pace, Karen Miller, Fran Krichek and Mimi Galgano

Chapter Five

High Points and Dead Ends

The West Islip Breast Cancer Coalition was only the *second* of the codified breast cancer grassroots advocacy groups to be established on Long Island. The *first* was one that many in the WIBCC knew well and, in fact, had participated in actively.

Before the mapping project, a number of them had attended a breast cancer support group in the early 1990s that was sponsored by the social work school at Adelphi University in Nassau County. Marie Quinn also attended the group.

A beautiful, statuesque woman in her early 40s, Marie was chairwoman of the guidance department at Wantagh High School. She was troubled by the fact that the chemotherapy she was receiving for breast cancer was the same "therapy" that her mother had received 20 years before. When her puzzlement turned to anger and then energy, Marie – who had always been completely apolitical – decided to start a new organization that had an aggressive political agenda. With her friend Fran Kritchek (also a breast cancer patient), Marie approached the influential director of the Adelphi program, Barbara Balaban.

Barbara was a seasoned veteran of social and political action. In addition to being at the forefront of the anti-Vietnam War movement in the 1960s, she and her psychiatrist husband, Al, were among

135

the founders of the first national organization for children with growth disorders, effectively introducing the treatment of human growth hormone to a public that had no idea that *anything* existed to treat young people who failed to grow at a normal rate.

With master's degrees in social work and counseling, as well as advanced certificates from prestigious programs in family and behavioral therapy, Balaban had worked as a crisis counselor and oncology social worker before she assumed the directorship of the Adelphi program in 1989. Aware of – and infuriated by – the lack of awareness that existed among elected officials and the general public about the widespread incidence of breast cancer on Long Island, and not at all shy about fighting the "powers-that-be," she seized upon Marie's idea with a vengeance, immediately setting up a meeting of community shakers and movers to implement a plan of action.

After a few sessions, the group created a name for their new organization, and on November 27, 1990, 1 in 9: The Long Island Breast Cancer Action Coalition was formally established – so named for the number of American women who would get breast cancer in their lifetimes. It took several months to set up the organization, determine the role of each person who would help make it work, round up corporate and political sponsors, and formulate plans for its first ambitious project – the first-ever rally for breast cancer awareness, to be held on October 23, 1991, on the steps of the Nassau County Supreme Courthouse, the same building that housed the regional offices of major TV, radio, and print journalists.

The rally generated a thunderstorm of recognition. An unprecedented number of invited politicians attended and, for the first time, spoke with passion and conviction about the plague of breast cancer on Long Island and what they planned to do about it.

The rally attracted an impressive 300 participants and the media were riveted by the large and dramatic 1 in 9 banner, the clusters of balloons (eight pink and one black), the tables that featured post-mastectomy prostheses and post-chemotherapy turbans, and a number of provocative placards featuring slogans such as "Breast Cancer is Unacceptable!" and "Too Many L.I. Women Are Dying of Breast Cancer!" and "Our Silence is Over!" – as well as those held by the young children of breast cancer survivors that said "I Want My Mom to Live!" and "Why is Breast Cancer Killing My Mother?"

The demonstration served as a high point in breast cancer advocacy and excited media people who, up to that point, had given the subject a low priority. As cameramen ran out of film and newsprint journalists scrounged desperately for extra pads of paper, the fledgling organization's members knew they had made a powerful impression. Having taken a page from the AIDS activists of the previous decade who were fed up with the sluggish response of health officials and legislators to the urgency of their plight, 1 in 9's members had put names and faces on the scourge of breast cancer, sacrificing their privacy to break the age-old taboo of never speaking aloud about the disease.

The evening news, on both local and New York City TV and radio stations, featured the rally in lead stories. Bold headlines in local and regional newspapers blared reports of the event.

"They got it!" Marie exclaimed in both amazement and delight. Yes, the media finally understood that each woman who attended the rally had changed her status from "victim" to "advocate."

The rally represented a dramatic turning point for the women in attendance and for those who read and heard about it and saw it on TV. Almost overnight, 1 in 9 took off like a rocket, establishing liaisons with politicians, mobilizing a speakers' bureau, and holding well-publicized and well-attended fund-raisers. Since the new coalition was housed at Adelphi, numerous of its support-group members and volunteers from its Breast Cancer Hotline joined 1 in 9 in helping to put the breast cancer issue "on the map."

Newspaper reporters soon found themselves interviewing women who were angry, not depressed. TV spots featured women who refused to speak about treatments and insisted instead on talking about finding a cure for the disease by demanding that their legislators enact laws that increased research funding. Ironically, given the deadly nature of the subject that members of 1 in 9 and Adelphi were discussing, it was a heady time.

In a matter of months, the members of 1 in 9 had "learned the ropes" of political involvement, realizing that the fight against the disease was as much about legislation and money as it was about treatments. Frustrated, even angry, that the first Long Island study had yielded no answers, they maintained a steady drumbeat of demands for a *new* Long Island study.

Their pleas were heard. With elections a little more than a year away, Long Island politicians were already gearing up. There were rumblings that Senator D'Amato, facing his third race for the Senate in what would become known as "The Year of the Woman," would be challenged by Brooklyn Congresswoman Elizabeth Holtzman, who was well known for her advocacy of women's issues.

In spite of the senator's effectiveness as a legislator and his increasing power in Washington, his stand against abortion alienated many women, and for most of his tenure he hadn't embraced the breast cancer issue. All that changed when he realized that Long Island activists were making breast cancer their number one issue.

Three months after the 1 in 9 rally, on January 31, 1992, Senator D'Amato announced that, as a result of an urgent request he had made to Dr. William L. Roper, the director of the federal Centers for Disease Control and Prevention in Atlanta, the CDC had agreed to conduct a study of environmental factors as the possible cause of breast cancer on Long Island. He also urged the Environmental Protection Agency to conduct its own separate study on Long Island. It was an astounding victory for Long Island's activists, proof positive that their efforts had paid off.

But the thrill was short-lived, as was just about every sign of progress in the one-step-forward/two-steps-back journey of the breast cancer activists. As months and then nearly a year elapsed and the conclusions of the CDC's study were not forthcoming, it became clear that important announcements and lofty promises were not always trustworthy.

The only thing the activists grew to trust was Senator D'Amato's commitment. From the day he came "on board," he never removed the pink breast cancer pin from his lapel, nor did he stop fighting for a new study.

The Kitchen Revolutionaries' mapping project began 10 months after the rally and seven months after the senator's announcement. When the project began, many of the West Islip women became aware that they couldn't fight for the various agendas of 1 in 9 and Adelphi *and* map their own community's incidence of breast cancer. But they thought that by working separately on different projects they would complement each other, providing a positive image and a wealth of substance to what was becoming the Long Island breast cancer "movement."

"It was like we were zooming along on an open highway," Lorraine said, "and all of a sudden we turned onto a dead-end street. If many of our members stayed with 1 in 9, our project would never get finished, but if they left 1 in 9 we'd be giving up other projects we believed in."

As it turned out – at least for a time – Adelphi's program, 1 in 9, and the WIBCC had so many identical interests that most of their members continued to participate in one another's activities.

A major effort took place just a month after the mapping project appeared on the front page of *Suffolk Life*. In a trip organized by Barbara Balaban, Lorraine and the women of the West Islip Breast Cancer Coalition, along with dozens of other activists boarded a bus to Washington, D.C., at four in the morning, to lobby members of Congress for research funds to find out why Long Island women had such a high rate of breast cancer. When they arrived back on Long Island at 11 o'clock that evening, the women were flush with victory, or at least hopeful that the promises they'd received from various legislators would be fulfilled.

The next month, on October 13, 1992, many of the same women – as well as hundreds of their supporters – attended the second annual breast cancer awareness rally at the Nassau County Courthouse. Broadway and television performer Phyllis Newman, who recently had been diagnosed with breast cancer, added "star power" to the event, and Matuschka, a New York City artist, stopped people in their tracks with her arresting graphics of a one-breasted woman, for which she, herself, had been the model.

Notably absent but very much in the minds and hearts of the attendees was Marie Quinn, the cofounder of 1 in 9. After being honored during Women's History Month the previous March, she had returned to her home, collapsed and died at the age of 48, having made a spectacular contribution to what would ultimately become a national breast cancer movement.

Marie's co-president, Fran Kritchek, spoke with passion at Marie's funeral, telling the audience of 300: "This is breast cancer month, but for women on Long Island, every month is breast cancer month." Although she was naturally soft-spoken, her message was atypically aggressive: "Politicians fund what they fear, and they don't fear breast cancer," she said, noting that "if prostate cancer or testicular cancer were the subjects, we'd see the kind of funding that women need for breast cancer."

Just a day after the rally, on October 14, Fran, Lorraine, Ginny Regnante, Barbara Balaban, and 1 in 9's Joan Flaumenbaum, among others, traveled back to Washington, D.C., to meet with the National Breast Cancer Coalition and, once again, to lobby their legislators. They were intent on presenting members of Congress with demands for a new Long Island breast cancer study and increased funding for breast cancer research. They were heartened that Senator D'Amato was on board to support the women as they pursued the NBCC's initiative to obtain $300 million from the Department of Defense. Arriving at his office, they sported long pink ribbons on their clothing inscribed with the words: "$300 Million More!" Their zeal shored up the senator's commitment to fight for the funding and they let him know that they expected that number would go even higher in the years to come.

When the women arrived in Washington, they were surprised to learn that a brief meeting had been arranged with a presidential candidate's wife, Hillary Clinton. Boarding a bus for Williamsburg,

Virginia, the women found themselves stranded when the bus broke down. Undaunted, they convinced a sheriff to escort them to the 15-minute meeting, which turned into a half-hour meeting in which the women regaled the candidate's wife with breast cancer statistics and the need for increased legislation, research, and research funding. To their satisfaction, Mrs. Clinton responded by saying, "We have to change the way the decision-making process in this country [is made]... I want your suggestions to be acted upon. If they're not, call me up – we want to do this right!"

Back in Washington, they joined thousands of women who had already swamped members of Congress with phone calls, letters, and telegrams and were now swarming through the halls of Congress to reinforce the urgent need for research funding. Their resoundingly successful trip ultimately led to over $400 million in new funds for breast cancer research.

Every Long Island advocate who made the trip returned to her home resolved to redouble her effort. By now – 10 months after Senator D'Amato's announcement of a new Long Island breast cancer study had yielded no plan of action from the CDC – every activist from every group was convinced that the breast cancer issue deserved front-burner status. While each organization pursued its individual goals, *all* of them began calling for a new study, and Lorraine's mapping project took on renewed urgency.

The WIBCC mailing had already been accomplished, thanks to the Revlon grant arranged by Congressman Tom Downey, and the return had been impressive, but it was not "the whole enchilada"

143

that the Kitchen Revolutionaries felt they needed to make the analysis of the study credible and irrefutable. They still needed additional funds for one more mailing.

Lorraine called Senator Johnson's office to ask about the grant she had spoken to him about and was told that it was "in the works" and would probably be forthcoming "in the near future," reassurances that sounded to her like "The check is in the mail."

She was impatient to move her project forward, but, exciting as it had been, it had also turned her home into a circus. While she continued to be irritated by the complaints of her brothers-in-law, the pressure to find an office was yet one more thing to worry about. She vowed to herself to keep an eye on real estate prospects and asked her son to do the same. But the main preoccupation of all the women in the WIBCC was the survey.

Yet, as unswerving as their commitment was to finishing the mapping project, life was making demands on many of the women, and there were days that only one or two managed to make it to Lorraine's house.

The end of 1992 was slow. But slow times and fast times, small glitches and large obstacles were familiar to the women, and they began to consider all of them a metaphor for the very subject they were investigating: dead-end streets – and the possible hazard they presented to women in West Islip.

"So what if *this* month is a dead end?" the ever-optimistic Ginny

Regnante said when progress seemed particularly sluggish. "That's what started us and that's what may lead us to answers." In a somewhat magical way of thinking, she and the rest of the women came to consider dead ends as the start of something big, even when "real life" threatened to undermine their optimism.

There were deaths of family members, colleagues, and friends with breast cancer, children with broken bones, and challenges such as college applications. There were Christmas and birthday presents to buy and vicious bouts of winter flu. But through it all they continued making good progress, although they knew that many months of work lay ahead.

Many of the WIBCC women worked at jobs where computers had become a way of life, and they often laughed at the primitive style of their data collection – file card by file card, Magic Marker stroke by Magic Marker stroke.

In stark contrast was the high-tech part of their effort, the e-mail transmissions that were pouring in to Lou Grasso's office, which he faithfully conveyed to the women; the radio interviews conducted by telephone, many reaching a national audience; and the TV appearances in the tri-state area of New York, New Jersey, and Connecticut, a large number of them beamed by satellite to other parts of the country.

It was gratifying to the women that their work was being recognized and increasingly legitimized by TV commentators and newspaper people. Most satisfying was the effect that coalition members had in inspiring the larger Long Island community through their frequent speaking engagements. In high school auditoriums packed to the rafters, in front of church and synagogue groups, at political rallies, and before the increasing number of community groups to which they were invited, the women's passion was contagious.

And their message was a call to arms: It's our cancer, our bodies, our futures, our lives, and maybe our deaths! We have a right to answers!

Their message was being heard. Among other signs of what they hoped would signal progress was the long-awaited CDC report that Senator D'Amato had asked for months before. Holding a press conference at the Mineola courthouse on January 7, 1993, the senator – surrounded by over two-dozen activists from Adelphi, 1 in 9, and the WIBCC – came out fighting, vilifying the CDC for "slipshod work."

Citing the contradictory conclusions of the federal agency's report – that much remained to be learned *and* that further study was not necessary – he said that the panel had "squandered a valuable opportunity to highlight the areas in need of further research."

"Instead of clarity and intelligence," D'Amato admonished the CDC, "we got contradiction and neglect." He called the report "a cover-up" and said the CDC had "missed the boat on the unknown risk factors that accounted for as much as 75 percent of all breast cancer occurrences on Long Island."

Calling once again for a new study, the senator vowed to his constituents that he wouldn't rest until the powers-that-be in Washington met his demands. The press conference energized the women, sending them back to their various projects with renewed vigor.

By March of 1993, the snows of winter had melted into spring, and the new season brought stunning news and affirmation to the activists that their voices had been heard: The U.S. House of Representatives had passed a bill directing the National Cancer Institute to conduct environmental studies of Long Island's high breast cancer rate!

While there was celebrating all around, the women were sophisticated enough about political matters to know that the bill still had to be passed by the Senate and signed by the president (both of which, months later, ultimately took place). In the meantime, there was work to be done.

A couple of weeks later, during Women's History Month, Lorraine joined renowned scientists, environmental activists, public officials, and women's groups in New York City at a meeting organized by the Women's Environmental Development Organization (WEDO), an international nonprofit organization that aimed to advance the role of women in policy-making. The goal of the conference, chaired by former Congresswoman Bella Abzug, was to explore the role that environmental contaminants *might* play in the rising incidence of breast cancer.

The invitation was one of many that Lorraine – as well as an increasing number of other breast cancer activists on Long Island – was eager to attend. All the women were fast learning that getting their own names in the public arena and rubbing elbows, so to speak, with prominent politicians and scientists were vital to keeping their demands for funding, research, and a new study both front and center of public awareness.

Ironically, the greater the number of prestigious invitations the women received, the more the competition among them increased. Instead of considering attendance at a science or political forum a boost to their own coalitions or to the entire grassroots movement, they looked on with anger and envy if any one of them was not included. With amazing rapidity, they had learned that saying, in essence, "I am woman – hear me roar!" was no longer enough. As each group – and often each individual – strived for prominence, photo ops, media attention, and access to the higher-ups, those precious invitations took on new urgency.

At the WEDO conference, Lorraine introduced herself to the flamboyant Ms. Abzug, who was wearing one of her trademark, equally flamboyant hats. Abzug praised the mapping project but remarked how shocked she was to learn about the many cases of breast cancer on Long Island, saying that she spent a lot of time each summer in Sag Harbor in the Hamptons and so hoped Lorraine's suspicions were wrong. Sadly, three months after the conference, she was diagnosed with breast cancer.

At the meeting, representatives from the American Cancer Society and the National Institutes of Health agreed that breast cancer had *not* reached "epidemic" proportions, a view that elicited plenty of dissent. To rousing cheers, Dr. Samuel Epstein, professor of occupational and environmental medicine at the University of Chicago and a leading cancer expert known for his outspoken criticism of the "cancer establishment," reiterated the claims he made in his 1978 book, *The Politics of Cancer*, that the National Cancer Institute and the American Cancer Society were culpable for losing the war against cancer because of their indifference to prevention, misleading claims, and pervasive conflicts of interest.

Another speaker was Devra Lee Davis, M.P.H., Ph.D., and Scholar-in-Residence at the National Research Council of the National Academy of Sciences in Washington, D.C. Dr. Davis was at the forefront of alerting the public to the potential dangers that estrogens played in increased rates of breast cancer. She told the audience that in addition to increased exposure to estrogens because of earlier periods, later menopause, and the use of birth control pills, fertility pills, and hormone replacement therapy, women also were exposed to the hormone through xenoestrogens, which were found in plant life and mimicked estrogen in the body.

Jay M. Gould, Ph.D., an epidemiologist, statistician, and prolific author who served on the science advisory board of the Environmental Protection Agency during the Carter administration, spoke of the epidemiological evidence that demonstrated the adverse health effects of low-level radiation. His message was echoed by Ernest Sternglass, Ph.D., another widely respected author and a professor of radiological physics at the University of Pittsburgh Medical School, whose research and testimony had played a role in President Kennedy's decision to sign the Partial Nuclear Test Ban Treaty.

Most arresting was the testimony of Mary S. Wolff, Ph.D., associate professor of community and preventive medicine and director of the division of environmental health sciences at the Mount Sinai Medical Center in New York, whose study about the effects of DDT had recently been published. Dr. Wolff found that women with the highest levels of DDT in their tissue were four times more at risk for breast cancer because the toxic chemical was stored in the fatty tissue of the breast and increased the amount of estrogen in the body. She said that breast milk contained more DDT residues than is allowed in milk cartons on grocery store shelves and that another source of the chemical came from pesticides that were routinely used on lawns.

The forum ended with the participants drafting a report for local and national politicians that included public-policy recommendations reflecting a greater commitment to women's health. Lorraine was elated to be a contributor to WEDO's policy statement and thrilled about the publicity the conference generated.

The day after the WEDO forum, before she had time to take a breath, Lorraine was back home working on the surveys. Real life, however, continued to intrude on the mapping project. There was the IRS deadline to meet, bothersome allergies to treat, electrical outages, flat tires, appliance breakdowns, and plain old bad moods. There were weddings, communions, bar and bat mitzvahs and wakes to attend, as well as vacations to take. And, for many of the women, chemotherapy and radiation treatments which Lorraine was undergoing at the time and their attendant side effects to deal with.

Yet, woven like a bright thread into the fabric of their daily lives was the ever-present – and very positive – interest of the media. Melba Tolliver, the anchor on Long Island's Cablevision network, News 12, interviewed Lorraine at length, and Christine Conniff Sheahan, the publisher and editor of *Networking*, the monthly news magazine she owned in Southampton, published article after article about the mapping project, as did the *Islip Bulletin* and numerous other newspapers, and Liz Tonis of *Suffolk Life* kept up her relentless coverage.

Each newscast and article generated increased local interest and support, but nothing like the flood of attention that occurred when Lorraine, Geri Barish and a number of other survivors and activists appeared on the cover of *Ms.* magazine, and after Lorraine was interviewed on CNN's *Eye to Eye* with Connie Chung and the mapping project was featured on ABC-TV's *Prime Time Live* with Diane Sawyer.

On Ms. Sawyer's program, Lorraine explained why breast cancer patients could no longer trust "the experts" and *had* to take matters into their own hands, she said, "The silence is over." The phrase reverberated in the hearts and minds of thousands upon thousands of viewers, many who called and wrote to Lorraine to say, "Yes! We agree!" Interestingly, many viewers heard the phrase as "The science is over," and they, too, agreed that "Science cannot be trusted, but we can trust your mapping project!" However they heard the sentence, dozens of people wanted to know how to map the incidence of cancer in their own communities and invited Lorraine to show them how.

Other members of the Kitchen Revolutionaries were interviewed as well, bringing the power of their own personalities and their perspectives on the breast cancer problem to the public. In addition, numerous women from 1 in 9, Adelphi, and a burgeoning number of new coalitions also enjoyed a lion's share of media attention, all of which served to give the Long Island breast cancer problem – and the many projects of the various groups – constant, high-profile exposure.

But neither celebrity nor the demands and arduousness of their personal or professional lives stopped the West Islip women from rousing themselves out of bed every morning to make their way to Lorraine's home, where they often punctuated the grim nature of the survey with rollicking humor. One of their daily breaks inevitably came when little Alyssa would cry to have her diaper changed. "Poo-poo time," one of the women would say, as the rest laughed out loud at this unlikely interruption of their science project.

Days and weeks flew by. As May rolled around, the women of the WIBCC felt chagrined at having been denied the opportunity to speak at a Nassau County breast cancer rally and were determined to establish what they hoped would become an annual rally in Suffolk County. Lorraine persuaded then-Suffolk County Executive Robert Gaffney to hold such a rally and ultimately served as keynote speaker in a speech she entitled "We Want to Know!"

Held on the steps of the imposing H. Lee Dennison building on May 6, 1993, the rally inspired Gaffney to institute the Suffolk County Breast Health Partnership – which helped underserved women to obtain mammogram screenings – under the directorship of longtime activist Joan Therese Hudson. In keeping with her support of "anything that helps women to fight the curse of this disease," Lorraine became a charter member.

By this time, it was clear to even the most casual onlooker that the work of the Long Island breast cancer coalitions had convinced an increasingly large number of people that the environment was somehow implicated in the rising rates of cancer. Dozens of forums were held, including a well-attended event at Adelphi at which representatives from the international organization Greenpeace, the Long Island–based Citizens Campaign for the Environment (CCE), and the New York State Public Interest Research Group (NYPIRG) regaled the audience with what Joan D'Argo of Greenpeace called "incontrovertible evidence" that organochlorines and thousands of other industrial chemicals were known to cause cancer and that "177 of them have been found in tissues, breast milk, semen, and the blood and breath of people in North America."

D'Argo also spoke about the chlorine bleaching process used in producing sanitary napkins, tampons, and disposable diapers, saying that the process left traces of dioxin, which was known to cause cancer, birth defects, miscarriages, and damage to the immune system. She urged the audience to follow the lead of English citizens who had waged a campaign of 50,000 letters to manufacturers and Parliament that – in six weeks – forced the manufacturers to switch to less-harmful oxygen-bleached paper.

Katherine Diecks from CCE told the rapt audience that the deep recharge areas of drinking water on Long Island were contaminated because organic substances were tested only four times a year, and hundreds of inactive hazardous sites and leaking underground storage tanks posed additional dangers to human health. And the audience gasped when Laurie Valeriano from NYPIRG reported that Grumman Aerospace, one of Long Island's major industries, had dumped over a million pounds of toxic substances into the soil over the years.

Present at the forum was Liz LoRusso of 1 in 9, a breast cancer patient and mother of two young children. Visibly suffering from – in fact almost debilitated by – the effects of chemotherapy, she carried a placard that said, "Mothers are Dying for Funding for Research." With great difficulty, she rose from her chair to express a statement that embodied the new mentality that had taken hold on Long Island since the rise of the advocacy movement and the mapping project: "Finally," she said, "people are beginning to see that breast cancer is not a woman's fault."

154

Indeed. The invitations that were pouring into the WIBCC gave ample evidence that those who issued them didn't blame women at all, that they too believed "something" in the environment accounted for the curse of breast cancer in the region.

The following months zoomed by with equal speed. As the summer of '93 passed – "like a blur," one woman said – the volunteers began to see light at the end of what had become a seemingly endless tunnel of work. At the end of September, they began talking about the great challenge that lay ahead of them: completing their work!

The work that lay before them took an unexpected and exciting turn when Lorraine received an invitation from Long Island Congressman Rick Lazio to attend a meeting with President Clinton at the White House. Lazio knew that she and a number of Long Island women had already planned a trip to the nation's capital for a meeting with the National Breast Cancer Coalition, their ultimate goal being to deliver to the president a mountain of letters generated by the NBCC's "Do the Write Thing" campaign, which lobbied for additional funding for breast cancer research.

Originally, the campaign had set out to collect 175,000 letters – one for each projected breast cancer diagnosis that year. But in an extraordinary demonstration of grassroots power, the campaign had generated 600,000 letters from around the country.

Rising at four in the morning, Lorraine and her friend Debra Gorstein, as well as Donna Ketcham, Maria Diorio, and Ginny

Regnante, boarded an Amtrak train for Washington, D.C., arriving at the Embassy Hotel to prepare for their historic meeting.

The meeting took place in the resplendent East Wing of the White House and was attended by First Lady Hillary Clinton; Donna Shalala, the secretary of Health and Human Services; Fran Visco, the founder and president of the National Breast Cancer Coalition; Matilda Cuomo, wife of New York State's Governor Mario Cuomo, and various other prominent personalities, as well as a number of members of other Long Island breast cancer coalitions, including 1 in 9 and representatives from Adelphi.

Lorraine was carrying the map rolled up under her arm but had it promptly confiscated by a White House security guard who assured her that he would show it to the President and return it to her after the meeting. President Clinton was well aware of the map, having learned of it on a CNN broadcast. He spoke movingly of the breast cancer issue and of his mother's battle with the disease, and he told the audience of the efforts Long Island women were making in collecting data. In closing, he said that he planned to support increased funding for breast cancer research – a pledge that every woman in the room planned to hold him to.

As if the meeting were not dizzying enough, Lorraine went straight from the White House to join thousands upon thousands of breast cancer activists who were spending the dazzlingly sunny day marching down Pennsylvania Avenue, banners aloft, to bring their plea for increased research funding and better legislation to

Capitol Hill and the public. Arm in arm with Geri Barish of 1 in 9 and a host of other Long Island activists, she marched with a phalanx of women who were chanting, "We're mad as hell and we're not going to take it anymore!"

At the end of October 1993, Lorraine was invited to join over 100 people at the Huntington Town Hall at one of the rare congressional subcommittee meetings held on Long Island. Senator D'Amato had called for the meeting – which was chaired by New York Senator Gary Ackerman – the point of which was to pressure the National Cancer Institute to make good on its promise to him months before to conduct a study to determine if the breast cancer incidence on Long Island was the result of elements in the environment. Congress had passed a provision calling for such a study but had failed to fund it.

D'Amato, who was also known as Senator Pothole because of his attention to the seemingly "small" things that troubled his constituents and the fierce battles he waged to redress their grievances, was serving his third six-year term, and his presence was both intimidating and effective. Although his campaigns for the Senate had received a torrent of bad publicity about his right-to-life stance, women who cared about breast cancer and the hundreds of thousands of people who were related to them or impressed by his fierce advocacy had come out in droves to vote for him.

Wearing a pink ribbon in his suit lapel, as he did every day – even at forums unrelated to breast cancer – he was the first speaker to rise and say his piece. Sporting a trim figure and a seemingly mild-mannered style, he smoothed back his thinning hair and adjusted his thin-rimmed glasses. Everyone in the room waited tensely for the man who some considered to be the most powerful man in the United States to proffer his opinion.

The breast cancer advocates were guardedly optimistic. The senator had already secured, in conjunction with Democratic Senator Tom Harkin from Iowa, $260 million to increase federal breast cancer research funding in fiscal year 1993, a 165 percent increase over the previous year. (Senator D'Amato was ultimately responsible for securing over $850 million for breast cancer research). D'Amato was also responsible for enacting a National Cancer Registries program to help researchers develop the exact statistical profiles needed to identify breast cancer patients.

Nevertheless, the women who sat in the audience, many of them missing a breast or even two, had been disappointed by the sluggish pace of legislation and sat with their fingers crossed, hoping and praying that the forum would not be yet another dead end.

The officials who sat on the dais were also guardedly optimistic, trusting that the behind-closed-doors discussions they had had with the senator would inspire him to moderate his advocacy and to take into consideration the budgetary and philosophical priorities of the National Cancer Institute, which were not always in sync with those of breast cancer activists.

All of them knew, however, that underneath the dese-dems-and-dose speaking style of the senator was a man who combined the combativeness and street-smarts savvy of his native Brooklyn with political instincts that had proved unerring in three hotly contested elections. His success seemed to lie not only in his tremendous grasp of complicated issues but also in his seemingly peculiar identification with the breast cancer issue.

On many occasions, the feisty 54-year-old senator had cited the issue as important to his 78-year-old mother, Antoinette, saying, "Mama is upset about this." He also never failed to mention his two daughters, Lisa and Lori, the wives his sons Christopher and Danny would one day have, and his numerous grandchildren, many of them female, as reasons he was battling for funding for breast cancer research.

In addition, D'Amato had met with a great number of Long Island breast cancer survivors and listened to their horrific stories. The ruts on the Long Island Expressway he was so famous for filling paled in comparison to the problems the women described, and when they made their needs known to him, particularly the need for a "real" study, he and his staff listened carefully and took copious notes.

Now, his constituents thought, the moment of truth had arrived. Sure enough, after smoothing out his necktie and clearing his throat, he launched into a blast at members of the Centers for Disease Control for failing to focus on the possible links between breast cancer and environmental contaminants. In language as clear as the crystal chandelier that hung overhead, he called for a coordinated federal effort to definitively establish a connection between the two.

Senator D'Amato's machete struck at "bureaucrats" in Washington as he reminded his audience that a woman who had lived in Nassau County for more than 40 years had a 72 percent greater risk of getting breast cancer than a women of the same age who had lived in the county for less than 20 years, and that a woman in Suffolk County was bound to die younger of the disease.

He blamed the lack of progress in the war against breast cancer on federal inaction in pursuing the connection between the disease and certain pesticides and other compounds (he mentioned the xenoestrogens that Dr. Davis had discussed at the WEDO conference, which mimic the effects of estrogen in the human body), and he challenged the panel to give him "one reason" not to give a green flag to a federal study.

"The Environmental Protection Agency is another federal agency that has gotten it wrong on breast cancer," the senator railed, accusing the agency of failing to develop a test system for screening pesticides, which had been used in huge amounts on Long Island potato farms, many of which were now divided into residential subdivisions. "These chemicals," he told his audience, "are from the same family of pesticides as DDT and other chemicals that are now suspected of possessing estrogen-mimicking properties."

There was no mistaking the senator's intent. His harsh and challenging remarks were further bolstered by the presence of Drs. Samuel Epstein and Devra Lee Davis, the former telling the panel that "We label food for cholesterol but we don't label for carcinogens, and I demand to know why."

Lorraine's voice rang out as well, telling the panel not only of her coalition's mapping efforts but also of the numerous grassroots groups that also were conducting mapping projects. "We're finding out things that 'big science' should be finding out," she said. "Long Island needs a new study!"

But it was the senator's challenge to the powers-that-be that the activists considered most important. After the meeting, they hugged and kissed each other, and only a week after D'Amato leveled his non-negotiable demands, the women took a train to Washington once again at four in the morning to visit his office and reinforce their support.

Bleary-eyed from sleeplessness, Lorraine and her colleagues arrived at his office only to learn from his science adviser, Scott Amrhein, that the senator was not there – he was fighting on the floor of the Senate for funding for the study, presenting his case with elaborate charts, printouts, and statistics.

A couple of weeks later, on November 8, 1993, the senator held a press conference to tell the country – and his constituents – that the officials at the National Cancer Institute had "committed" to spending several million dollars for a federal study of breast cancer and the environment on Long Island. The study, he explained, was to be authorized by the National Institutes of Health Revitalization Act, which had just been passed (and is now a public law) and to be conducted jointly by the NCI and the National Institute of Environmental Health Sciences. Its goal: to pinpoint precisely the role that pesticides and other environmental factors such as hazardous wastes, pollution, and electromagnetic fields from power lines played in Long Island's high breast cancer rates.

The NCI's decision was momentous. Never before had such a comprehensive and costly study been conducted. While the agency never admitted as much – at least at the time – those who had been following the ever-widening breast cancer movement on Long Island, including a number of influential members of the media, acknowledged that it was the mapping project of the Kitchen Revolutionaries that had played a key role in motivating the venerable institution to make its landmark decision.

Lorraine had always been confident that D'Amato would "deliver the goods." She had known him when he had served, years before, as the Supervisor for the Town of Hempstead in Nassau County and remembered that her politically active brother-in-law, Anthony Pace, along with Republican leader Anthony Prudenti, were the first political leaders to endorse D'Amato's bid for U.S. Senator in 1980. Since that time, she had seen him "in action," always fighting like a bulldog for the people he represented.

However, the perception that the WIBCC had been such a primary influence in the NCI's decision also contributed significantly to the internecine battles and dissension among activists that would grow as the months and years elapsed.

In truth, it was not the WIBCC's mapping project *alone* that forced the NCI to take action. From the day the project was first written about in the *Times* in July of 1992 and the survey published in *Suffolk Life* the following month, calls had poured into the West Islip group from community activists eager to translate Lorraine's idea into action.

Barbara Masry and Linda Ronn from the affluent North Shore of Long Island invited Lorraine to speak before their newly founded Great Neck Breast Cancer Coalition to teach them how to map their own community. Their coalition went on to institute a quilt-of-hope project and a lecture series in which prominent doctors and scientists spoke about the latest advances in breast cancer diagnosis and treatment to increasingly large audiences.

Another early caller was Karen Miller, who founded the Huntington Breast Cancer Coalition in 1993 with her friends Lynn Kotler, Anne Predun, and Mary Mohrman. Diagnosed with the disease in her early 40s, Karen's call was, again, to learn how to set up a mapping project in her community of 68,000 people. A trailblazer herself, she had been a participant in the Adelphi breast cancer support program and an early member of 1 in 9, but was fed up with the battles of the breast cancer advocates she was working with and wanted to strike out on her own. Lorraine advised Karen to "start small" with only one or two neighborhoods, but Karen insisted on mapping the entire community and, to this day, calls the project a "work in progress."

Karen went on to institute the "I Am Fed Naturally" UN-Pesticide Lawn Flag, a campaign that encourages homeowners to eliminate toxic chemicals on their property and promotes alternative methods of ground maintenance. Her coalition also started a breast-awareness training program (B.A.T.) to teach young women to become comfortable with the concept of breast health. And she was only one of two women (the other was Martha Rogers from the South Fork Breast Health Coalition) that the NCI selected from Long Island to be a Peer Reviewer Community Representative for its study.

These mapping projects, none of which had been completed or analyzed, as well as the unceasing drumbeat of advocacy from 1 in 9, Adelphi, and numerous other coalitions, were taking place when the NCI finally decided to begin its study in November of 1994. Their very existence, and the possibility that mere lay people would reveal information that would embarrass "the experts," had pressured the NCI to, as Ginny Regnante remarked, "come up with some answers."

Other people wanted answers as well. In 1994, Lorraine received a phone call from Francine Levian and Chris Mason of Marin County, California, a community that had the frightening distinction of having the highest breast cancer incidence in the world. They asked her if she could help them map their own community. Within weeks, Lorraine and John, along with Dr. Grimson and his wife, were on a plane to California. John explained the legal aspects of a mapping project, while Dr. Grimson detailed the ways in which they could create an accurate map. Francine and Chris went on to form the Marin County Breast Health Watch, which continues to thrive to this day, receiving major funding for research into the environment and its links to breast cancer.

When the NCI study was announced, Lorraine was relieved but also anxious that the mapping project had not been completed. Holding up its completion was the money she needed for the last mailing. The day after Senator D'Amato's announcement, she once again called State Senator Johnson's office. This time, he called her back immediately to say that he and Senator Caesar Trunzo, another Republican state senator from Long Island, had secured a grant for the WIBCC.

And not just any grant, but $80,000!

Lorraine was beside herself, tripping over her words to thank the senator and to let him know how important his and Senator Trunzo's belief in the project was to her and to all of the women on Long Island. She was too excited to listen to the details. All she knew, as she told the women who had worked with her for the past 16 months, was that they had finally "reached the light."

As it turned out, a small part of the grant was for the research project and a larger portion for a new home for the WIBCC. The grant was deposited in Stony Brook's account, with $20,000 earmarked for Dr. Grimson's analysis of the study. The rest of the money was deposited in the coalition's account to be used for office space, administrative help, a breast cancer awareness walkathon that was planned to generate further publicity for the project, and, most pressing, the last mailing – which was completed in just a week!

Lorraine called Good Samaritan Hospital to tell Ted Shiebler about the large state grant and to say that the WIBCC could now pay for office space at Good Sam – if it was available. After presenting her case to the hospital administration and navigating through what appeared to be the kind of bureaucratic snafus that could only be interpreted as more dead ends, Lorraine received a call from Shiebler a few weeks later saying that, yes, the coalition had a new home!

In January of 1994, 17 months after the Kitchen Revolutionaries started their mapping project – and, in fact, after their work was completed – the coalition moved into its own office on the main floor of the Baxter Pavilion in Good Samaritan Hospital on Montauk Highway in West Islip. Everyone was elated – especially Lorraine's neighbors!

The women had done such an expert job in organizing the original data that they left the project a brilliant legacy, one that would be used in the years to come to collate and pinpoint cases of cancer in towns and cities throughout the country, and, as it turned out, throughout the world.

Their primitive tools were pens, pencils, paper, handheld calculators, three-by-five cards, and Magic Markers, not the hi-tech computers and sophisticated data-analysis techniques that would ultimately make sense of their work.

In addition to reaching numerous high points of progress and exhilaration, the Kitchen Revolutionaries had encountered formidable obstacles and demoralizing dead ends. But the ardent commitment and great personal sacrifice they brought to their work was the stuff that computers and scientists cannot measure. Ultimately they spearheaded a worldwide movement of grassroots advocacy that changed the way doctors and scientists and the general public thought about breast cancer.

By *not* believing what the "experts" had to say, they had charted an authentic epidemiological map – sipping coffee, munching on bagels, and changing little Alyssa's diapers in the process. By so doing, they inspired the National Cancer Institute – among the most powerful health organizations in the United States and, in fact, the world – to take notice and to find formidable amounts of money to conduct on Long Island the largest epidemiological study in its history, that of the possible relationship between breast cancer and the environment.

Chapter Six

The Ripple Effect

Throwing a pebble into a body of water and watching the ripples and waves it creates seems to fascinate everyone, both those who hurl the tiny object and those who simply observe its effect. A stone, of course, creates a larger eddy, and a rock a whirlpool.

No doubt part of this fascination stems from the sheer visual delight of seeing the swirling circles of water fanning out in almost perfect symmetry. But I suspect that the power of this simple act is so universally appealing – and symbolic – because it affords the thrower a feeling of immense, albeit fleeting, power: *My* act has altered the movement of the ocean! (Or river or brook or even bathwater!)

When Lorraine began her mapping project in 1992, she unwittingly threw a boulder into the waters of breast cancer activism on Long Island – waters that already were roiling with activity.

At the time, increasing numbers of journalists had begun to address the subject with increasing aggressiveness. Barbara Balaban, the director of the Adelphi University breast cancer support program, had applied for and obtained a grant to set up a statewide toll-free "hotline" number. Marie Quinn and Fran Kritchek had founded 1 in 9, the first political action coalition in the region. Politicians were already making breast cancer a

168

priority and enacting legislation to improve care and access and increase research funding.

It was therefore inevitable that the surging waves the mapping project produced would splash up against the other activist projects, sometimes advantageously, other times in more negative ways. At the outset of the project, the huge swells of publicity the project generated were far-reaching, inspiring untold numbers of Long Island's women to applaud and emulate the West Islip group's efforts. But as the project progressed, the ripples and waves that might have united the activists into a cohesive force turned into rivalries of flood-like proportions.

However, the "bad stuff," as Lorraine called it, evolved slowly and was not dramatically apparent during the 17 months of the WIBCC's mapping effort, although hints of discontent had already begun to emerge by the time the project was completed in December of 1993. The previous month had been filled with stunning progress: a commitment by the National Cancer Institute to conduct a new Long Island study and an $80,000 grant to the WIBCC that facilitated the final mailing of the survey to West Islip residents.

At the very same time, other groups on Long Island were making a significant mark. On November 15-16, 1993, 1 in 9 co-sponsored a first-of-its-kind scientific forum with Adelphi: "Breast Cancer and the Environment – What We Know, What We Don't Know, What We Need to Know." The symposium was convened to reinforce to both activists and the public alike that, in spite of the naysayers, skeptics and state-employed scientists who continued to play down environmental causes of breast cancer, some of the world's most prominent researchers and clinicians disagreed.

The meeting featured 25 important scientists from around the world – each of whom waived an honorarium – and many hundreds of spectators, including political figures and their representatives as well as media people, who covered the event with avid curiosity and a blitz of newsprint and TV coverage.

The symposium was co-chaired by breast cancer surgeon Dr. Susan Love, director of the UCLA Breast Cancer Center in Los Angeles, internationally recognized author and a key founder, with breast cancer patient and lawyer Fran Visco, of the National Breast Cancer Coalition, and Dr. Devra Lee Davis, a cancer researcher and senior adviser to the Assistant Secretary of Health and Human Services at the National Academy of Sciences.

Dr. Love told the rapt audience, "The breast cancer puzzle is of enormous complexity. We don't even have a clue as to what the risk factors are. In the past, we focused on individuals and what they may have been doing to bring about breast cancer; now we must focus on our society and how it is causing breast cancer. Right now we have more questions than answers…in research, it's more important to be lucky than to be smart."

Dr. Jay Gould, of the Radiation and Public Health Project, explained to the audience the effect that low doses of radiation emissions had on lowering the immune system and thereby making people more susceptible to cancer. Between 1950 and 1965, he said, the Long Island–based Brookhaven National Laboratory was one of the three largest emitters of nuclear fission products in the country, and "this fact should force the authorities to test the radioactivity in drinking water in Nassau and Suffolk" because "it would explain why Long Island has so much cancer."

Louise Brinton, M.P.H., Ph.D., from the National Institutes of Health, spoke about the provocative but inconclusive studies pointing to the relationship between breast cancer and high-fat diets, ending her speech with the caveat "but we need more research." Lenore Kohlmeier, Ph.D., from the Department of Epidemiology at the University of North Carolina, spoke about the geographic variation in breast cancer rates between the U.S. and countries such as Japan and China, where women don't take birth control pills or post-menopausal estrogens.

When Daniel Wattenberg, Ph.D., an epidemiologist at the Environmental and Occupational Health Sciences Institute in Piscataway, New Jersey, was asked if Long Island was a good place to study breast cancer, he responded, "Unfortunately, it is a very good place."

Speaker after speaker illuminated the audience about the possible relationship of breast cancer to organochlorines, ambient air, pesticides, drinking water, radioactivity, landfills, electromagnetic fields, motor exhaust, and estrogen exposure. Frightening as the information was, the symposium was a resounding success, the activists having managed to assemble – for the first time ever

– the most authoritative voices in breast cancer treatment and research in the world.

It was one thing to read about their work in abbreviated versions, to discuss this or that finding in support groups, and to bring the information to the attention of doctors, politicians, and reporters. But to "see" the scientists in the flesh, to hear their voices, to perceive their commitment and concern – this experience enlivened the breast cancer activists on Long Island and inflamed the media.

The effect rippled all the way to Washington, D.C. By the following week, Dr. Samuel Broder, the director of the National Cancer Institute, agreed to meet with Geri Barish and Fran Kritchek, 1 in 9's co-presidents, to talk about ways in which the upcoming NCI study should be conducted. Their meeting received even more media attention and served to establish 1 in 9 as a prominent leader in what Geri Barish called "the fight that none of us can afford to lose."

Many of the Kitchen Revolutionaries attended the symposium and contributed to the question-and-answer discussion that followed the presentations. But even as they stood up to make their views – and their mapping project – known, they were preoccupied with the stunning events taking place in their own neck of the woods.

The stalwarts who stayed to the end, attending the mapping project almost every day for – at that time – 15 months, knew that their work was drawing to a close. Just three weeks after the Adelphi symposium – right before Christmas – their work was done. The data had been collected, the door-to-door sojourns had ended, the map had been marked and sent to Roger Grimson at Stony Brook to analyze, and the move to an office of their own at Good Sam had already begun.

To many of the women, the end of the project and the impending move to Good Sam was disconcerting and sad. The project had provided many of them with a raison-d'être, a way to translate their fear and anxiety and rage into concrete action. On the other hand, some of the women said they were relieved to finally get their lives back. Lorraine never missed a beat. She knew that the office represented the most important phase of the project, and she was champing at the bit to get going.

Her first priority was setting up the office, and she enlisted her sons to help her haul file cabinets, desks, plants, and pictures from her home and real estate office to her new digs. Fredi O'Connor and Pat Licata were paid as secretaries from the grant money to enter new data into the computer, "woman" the phones, start a WIBCC newsletter, field media questions, and set up interviews. Lorraine also purchased a fax machine and office supplies, happily accepted the donation of a computer, and managed to negotiate a bulk-rate mailing discount from Good Sam for any future mailings.

But to the reporters who had been hovering over every aspect of the project for months on end, the subject now became *when* the data would be analyzed. Lorraine was the primary target of this and other questions, and she found herself fielding dozens of media interviews while, at the same time, trying to set up, direct, coordinate, and generally run the WIBCC's new office.

It wasn't easy. She felt that she owed the media answers because she was grateful that so many reporters in local, regional, and national outlets had followed the story of the mapping project with such interest and support. When *Australia's 60 Minutes* called to interview her for a feature broadcast, she put on her "media hat" and appeared relaxed, but she wasn't. As one of the few "hands on" people to move the project from her home to Good Sam, every minute away from her new headquarters rattled her nerves.

In many instances she found herself cutting interviews short in order to run back to her new office. The one genuinely relaxed interview she experienced was with Osha Davidson, a writer from *Woman's Day*, probably because she was a fan of the magazine and felt that she identified with its readers – and that they would identify with her. And they did.

It wasn't only media pressure that spurred the project on. From the time the original survey was published, dozens of women had called Lorraine to say that the questionnaire was so "scary" that they had gone to get a mammogram – some for the first time – only to find that they had breast cancer! Of all the feedback she received, this was the most horrifying.

In a strange way, however, it was also encouraging. In her mind, the survey had become not only a way to find out if there were clusters of breast cancer in West Islip but also a way to spur, urge, or scare women into getting mammograms and perhaps saving their own lives.

At the same time, Lorraine was trying to deal with the profound changes that were taking place as the Kitchen Revolutionaries, emboldened and liberated by the $80,000 grant, decided that they wanted more control over the direction of the WIBCC. Underneath a veneer of good will were rumblings of discontent that would grow louder and more persistent as the weeks elapsed.

While she considered all the women her good friends, Lorraine knew that the strain of unfriendliness she detected was not in her imagination. The women were now powerful advocates and media celebrities in their own right, accustomed to being asked what they thought and felt about the general subject of breast cancer and about Long Island's problems in particular, and they believed that the decisions that came out of their new office should be by consensus, not determined unilaterally by Lorraine.

Lorraine was upset and confused by the increasing opposition she faced from her Kitchen Cabinet. She didn't understand it and wouldn't for many years, but there was simply no time to analyze or dwell on it. She and Fredi and Pat had already started to work – day and night – on establishing their new office.

Right from the beginning, however, there were problems that, as always, were interspersed with rays of light. The same month that the Good Sam office of the WIBCC was established, Lorraine's nonstop busyness was compounded by a family celebration and the lure of an offer she couldn't refuse. The celebration was for Donna Ketcham's engagement to John Jr. From their first meeting years before to their working together in John's real estate office to their impassioned work on the mapping project, Donna and Lorraine had "bonded" in so many ways that the engagement was, as Lorraine described it, "every mother's dream."

The enticing offer was from Stony Brook University to be the first breast health education "expert" they had ever hired, a job that involved community outreach and public education – exactly what she had been doing for the previous two years.

"They're paying me for this!" she crowed to her husband in disbelief. "And giving me an office and a secretary and a budget and a forum!" Again she thought of Elmer Gantry. She and he were both evangelists, she mused, "but his message was fake and my message is real." The opportunity was irresistible, and she hesitated not a millisecond before saying yes.

At the same time, a piece of unfinished WIBCC business would reveal the chasm developing between Lorraine and the other women in the organization, the issue being a WIBCC fund-raiser that had been in the planning stages for the previous two months. When every detail had been worked out and only the invitations remained to be mailed, a conflict arose as to where the funds should be allocated. All of the other women chose Good Sam, as a tribute to the project's new home and also to the hospital's new Breast Health Center. But Lorraine, knowing that the most important part of the survey – its scientific analysis – was about to begin, chose Stony Brook.

To call the conflict a mere disagreement would be to minimize its antagonistic nature, and its effects. So immovable were both parties that the fund-raiser hit a dead end. It fizzled into thin air.

Then there was the matter of fee-for-service. John Pace, who had provided his legal expertise and services on a voluntary basis to the mapping project from its inception, informed the group that he planned to charge a nominal fee for yet another piece of legal work, copyrighting the map. Bristling at what they considered an unreasonable change of heart, the women proceeded to hire a new lawyer for the WIBCC.

Another bone of contention arose when the women suspected that they were not being told about the many calls Lorraine was receiving at her home regarding speaking engagements, and that they were being excluded from many of the public statements and policy decisions she was issuing.

Particularly angry about these goings-on was Ginny Regnante, who felt that Lorraine wasn't "playing fair." A robust, full-figured woman with a ready laugh, Ginny had raised five children with her Italian husband, and she attributed Lorraine's "power grab" to her longtime marriage to an Italian patriarch.

"It's not easy being a nice Irish girl and marrying a guy who likes to call all the shots," she said. "When Lorraine finally got some power in her life, even though that power came from the horrible fact of having breast cancer, she liked it and she didn't want to give it up. And who would?"

Ginny and several other women in the West Islip coalition and in the other groups that were springing up everywhere on the Island and working on identical or similar issues felt that Lorraine was "grabbing all the attention." Some resented her speaking about clusters as if they actually existed, in essence diminishing their efforts to find out through scientific inquiry whether, in fact, they *did* exist.

"There are times you have to follow people who are smarter than you," said Ginny, one of the most outspoken critics of Lorraine's style of leadership, "and put your ego in your back pocket." She didn't think that Lorraine's ego was anywhere near her back pocket, but she continued to accept her as the leader of the WIBCC until the final straw in the growing schism occurred when Lorraine was asked to help develop a breast-health center at Stony Brook and wanted to bring the map with her to make her presentation.

The remaining members of the WIBCC had other ideas and acted on them, resulting in what would become a longtime "property" dispute. Without Lorraine's knowledge, Ginny had the map copyrighted as the legal property of the WIBCC. The group's original incorporation certificate in 1992 listed Lorraine as president and Ginny as vice president, but Ginny felt that the map represented the work and was the property of all the women who had labored over it for 17 months – that "it was larger and more significant than one person."

"This was not an individual effort," she told everyone who questioned the copyright. "This was the work of our coalition."

Lorraine was furious – and wounded – by what she perceived as a mutiny. She also saw the handwriting on the wall when Ginny told her that she "couldn't serve two masters" – in other words, she couldn't work for the university and also be a spokeswoman for the WIBCC, the agendas of which were often quite disparate.

While the women enjoyed the support of politicians and various local businesses that helped them with their fund-raisers, they still believed that their relationships had "no strings." The university, on the other hand, had community and political ties that they thought had the potential for conflicts of interest. More important, they thought that one of their main goals – to prevent some forms of breast cancer by eliminating carcinogenic chemicals from the environment – was more aggressive and therefore more likely to yield results than the university's goal of conducting laborious academic research that often tended to discredit – or at least cast doubt on – the "theories" of the women.

In spite of the tension, Lorraine continued her work with the WIBCC, striking an agreement with the coalition that her last day would be March 1, 1994. While she knew that her new job at the university would offer her a golden opportunity to educate huge numbers of people, she was still committed to "grassroots" outreach and feared that losing her affiliation with the WIBCC would cut her off from ordinary women who needed information and support.

Pondering the problem over a cup of soothing raspberry tea in her kitchen one Saturday morning, she had a brainstorm – yet another irresistible acronym: BC HELP (Breast Cancer Help: A Healthy Environment for a Living Planet). Without missing a beat, John Pace did the paperwork (pro bono, of course) that resulted in the incorporation of the new organization.

In order for her not to appear to be "serving two masters," Lorraine called upon her old friend and parish priest, Father Thomas V. Arnao of the Diocese of Rockville Centre, to be the director of BC HELP. In practically no time at all, she established a board of directors that included, among others, her oncologist Dr. Michael Feinstein; her radiation oncologist Dr. Allen G. Meek; her biking companion Roger Ryan; her administrative assistant at Stony Brook, Donna Cirincione; Maria Diorio, an original Kitchen Revolutionary; the Town of Islip Town Clerk, Joan Johnson; Carmen Imbo (who succumbed to breast cancer while serving on the board); Bea DeLizio, Maryann Fox, Antoinette Castiglio-Falciano, Alex Fezza, and her good friend Debra Gorstein. Additionally, while Breast Cancer HELP paid for normal expenses, John Pace, once again, volunteered to serve as the organization's attorney, waiving any and all legal fees.

Later members included Rick Shalvoy, a former lifeguard who gained notoriety on Long Island for honoring a friend who died of breast cancer by rowing a boat every summer around Long Island, some 300 miles, to raise funds for and awareness about the disease. There was John Zaher, a young man whose mother had died of breast cancer and who ultimately did public relations work for the organization. There was also Islip Town Councilwoman Pam Greene, who was more than willing to discuss Lorraine's idea for the first-ever breast cancer walk in Suffolk County. When the idea fell through, Lorraine presented it to Gloria Rocchio, then-director of The Stony Brook Fund, and Deborah Schreifels, of the community-relations department at Stony Brook Hospital.

Within months, "A Walk for Beauty in a Beautiful Place" became a reality as an encompassing grassroots effort that included the entire Stony Brook community, as well as its schools and scouting troops. Dozens of volunteers enhanced the effort, including Lorraine's son Greg, who was called upon to rise at four in the morning to fill in when the scheduled disc jockey cancelled at the last minute. By day's end, thousands of dollars had been raised for The Unique Boutique, which to this day provides – at no charge – wigs, prostheses, turbans and other accessories to women with breast cancer.

But the name BC HELP didn't last very long, as Lorraine realized that not everyone "in that great big public out there" recognized that BC stood for breast cancer. With her husband John getting all the legal papers in order, she promptly changed the name of the organization to Breast Cancer Help, Inc.

One day, a patient of Lorraine's radiation oncologist, Dr. Meek, showed up at a meeting of BC HELP. The doctor had told her that the organization would be a good place for her to translate her feelings of helplessness into action. As it happened, Diane Sackett Nannery didn't feel helpless. When she was diagnosed with breast cancer in her early 40s, the stunningly attractive self-described "health nut" felt enraged.

Even before her surgery, the formerly apolitical postal employee pored over every available piece of information about the disease, focusing on a relatively obscure side effect, lymphedema, a swelling that results from damage to the lymphatic system during surgery or chemotherapy and radiation treatments and is characterized by hugely swollen arms or legs, among other parts of the body.

The more she learned about the condition, the more it occurred to Diane that the chronic, lifelong malady might be avoided if hospital personnel forewarned patients about the potential danger of triggering lymphedema by having blood pressure readings, injections, and intravenous lines on the side of the body on which the surgery was performed. Drawing inspiration from the red wristband placed on patients who are allergic to medications, she thought that a pink wristband would serve a similar purpose for lymphedema.

Shortly after her surgery and while struggling through chemotherapy treatments, she sat down at her kitchen table and began writing in longhand to the nursing departments of local and regional hospitals, trying to convince them to institute her idea for a "pink wristband" policy. The idea caught on, soon spreading like wildfire to hospitals throughout the country and ultimately being embraced by the San Francisco-based National Lymphedema Network.

On a mission to raise society's consciousness and research monies for breast cancer, Diane began writing articles for the Postal Service newsletter, a publication that reached 750,000 postal employees nationwide. With the support and assistance of Breast Cancer HELP, she also spearheaded a successful drive for the issuance of the first-ever Breast Cancer Awareness postage stamp. She received a big boost for the project when Lorraine introduced her to Long Island Congressman Michael Forbes, who sat on a congressional committee involved with postal affairs. Forbes, who was aware of the AIDS stamp and thought a breast cancer stamp would be equally appropriate, wrote a letter to his colleagues supporting the project. The final design of the stamp was painted by Donna Ketcham Pace, while she was in early labor with Lorraine's first grandchild!

Lorraine worked side-by-side with Diane on the stamp issue, often introducing her to the powers-that-be, for instance Congressman Peter King, long an advocate of breast cancer issues, who immediately started a petition for the stamp in the House of Representatives, encouraging all of its members to sign on. Senator D'Amato did the same in the Senate.

Diane, who was vice president of Breast Cancer Help, Inc., also spearheaded "Give a Gift to Breast Cancer" check-off on the New York state income tax form. She told Lorraine that she had noticed a check-off box on her father-in-law's tax return form and wondered why the same couldn't appear on all state tax returns to allow residents and businesses to donate any whole dollar amount to breast cancer research and education.

Lorraine promptly arranged for her and Diane to meet with State Senator Owen Johnson, who immediately embraced the idea. Johnson then called his colleague, State Senator Charles Fuschillo, to work with him on the design and introduction of the bill in the state senate. The bill passed the Senate and Assembly, allowing all New York state residents to check "Give a Gift to Breast Cancer" on their tax returns. Subsequently, Lorraine, representing Breast Cancer Help, and Geri Barish, representing 1 in 9, supported legislation introduced by Assemblyman Steve Englebright to authorize the state to provide a dollar-for-dollar match for each contribution made to the fund.

Several months after her surgery, Diane was horrified to discover that *she* had lymphedema. Undaunted, she went on to coauthor a book about lymphedema (with the author of this book) for both doctors and patients.

With BC HELP in place, Lorraine continued her work with the West Islip group, but during her remaining months the atmosphere was permeated with contentiousness and ill will.

Shortly before Lorraine's day of departure arrived, Ginny Regnante (who had become the coalition's new president) and the other members of the group were called to a hastily scheduled eight p.m. meeting at Good Sam to meet with legislative aides from the offices of State Senators Owen Johnson and Caesar Trunzo. To their shock and stupefaction, they were told that the meeting was to challenge their authority to oversee the $80,000 that an "anonymous source" said they were spending "frivolously."

Through two hours of grueling questioning, the women presented their case, documenting each expenditure with receipts, correspondence, and the dates and times of their activities. Grimly, their interrogators thanked them for their time and said they'd be "getting back" to them within a week. Exactly one week later, the WIBCC members were told that they had answered all the questions satisfactorily and that they would remain the overseers of the grant.

The women believed that the whole unpleasant affair had been set up by Lorraine, and they felt betrayed – and enraged. But that is not where their enmity stopped. In short order, they received a demand from Stony Brook to send all of the $20,000 earmarked for Dr. Grimson's analysis of the data to the university – up front. This time, however, the women didn't depend on their own testimony to fight the order.

They hired the Suffolk County law practice of Siben & Siben to represent them and to insist that the money be sent to Dr. Grimson in increments; i.e., with each analysis report of the data, a payment would be made. Again, their wishes prevailed. In fact, the grant money was sent to the Stony Brook Research Fund, and Dr. Grimson never received a penny – his work was completely pro bono!

Relieved at getting what Ginny Regnante called "old business" out of the way, the WIBCC accelerated its efforts to track the responses the coalition had received – and was still receiving – on the computer system in their new office at Good Sam.

By March of 1994, Lorraine was out. Out of the coalition she had founded. Out of Good Sam. Out of the original copyright to her map. And out of touch with some of the women with whom she had spent nearly every day from August of 1992 to January of 1994.

But she was "in" at her new and exciting job at Stony Brook, in with the media, in with BC HELP, and in with other less glamorous things such as cancer checkups. In less than two years, she had fought depression, suffered through radiation and chemotherapy treatments, initiated an unprecedented mapping project, been hired for a prestigious job at a highly regarded university medical center, and founded two organizations.

No longer perceived as simply "a nice woman who sold real estate," she had become a ferocious advocate for breast cancer research and a powerful and influential force in the "politics of breast cancer." She had overcome dozens of dead ends with a cool head, a soft-spoken voice, and a resolute belief in her cause.

She also had amassed a huge file of prospective supporters – "fans," she called them – and when she went public with BC HELP, donations from both anonymous and known donors poured in, as did a flood of invitations to speak on Long Island. Although Lorraine was preoccupied with her new job, she felt that "spreading the word" by continuing to instruct other communities in how to start their own mapping projects would reinforce to the National Cancer Institute the importance of the study to which they had committed.

Mobilizing energies she didn't know she had, she plunged into her three "full-time" jobs: setting up BC HELP, working at her advocacy position at Stony Brook, and addressing the groups that invited her to speak. Maintaining her home, being a wife and mother, and attending to her own needs had become "part-time" jobs.

Her first engagement as a representative of her new organization was in Brentwood, where over two dozen women asked Lorraine how to set up their own grassroots breast cancer group and map their communities. By the end of the evening, the Brentwood-Bayshore Breast Cancer Coalition was established, and Lorraine donated nearly half of BC HELP's funds to help set up a mapping project in a minority area, which was overseen by the group's vice president, Marcia Clopton. Elsa Ford, a longtime activist in environmental issues, became president of the new coalition and would go on to become a prominent voice in breast cancer advocacy in the years to come.

Lorraine was well aware of and grateful for the comfortable circumstances in which she lived and of the instant access her economic comfort gave her to the best medical care – months of misdiagnoses notwithstanding. As she learned more and more about breast cancer, the stark disparity between white women and black women in early diagnosis, treatment, and prognosis startled her.

She knew that "making a difference" in women's lives meant in *all* women's lives, and she committed BC HELP to leading the charge, scheduling her next speaking engagement in a minority area in the town of Coram. By the end of the evening, a unified and passionate group of women had formed the Coram Breast Cancer Coalition, creating another ripple in the waters of breast cancer activism.

Charged by the enthusiastic receptions she received, Lorraine set her sights on the South Fork – East Hampton, Bridgehampton, Southampton, and other upscale areas where conversations run to Ralph Lauren and Donna Karan, art shows, and movie stars, and hardly ever to cancer. But the South Fork had a well-kept secret: the incidence of breast cancer in the region was the highest on Long Island, with 143 women out of 100,000 getting the disease.

Susan Roden and Martha Rogers founded the South Fork Breast Health Coalition and were hell-bent on getting answers, ultimately obtaining a $100,000 grant for a mapping project that ended up, years later, revealing another horrifying fact: the women getting breast cancer in this glamorous setting were younger than women in other parts of the country. In fact, incidence of the disease in women under the age of 54 was 60 percent higher than the Suffolk County average.

Lorraine received a call from Stony Brook, asking if she would speak to African-American women in Copiague. Her speech, emphasizing access to medical care and finding answers, enlivened the group's leader, Linda Hart, and in short order yet another coalition had been born: Sisters for Sisters with Breast Cancer.

As she stood before group after group, it was more apparent than ever to Lorraine that breast cancer was an equal-opportunity disease. It didn't matter what a woman's race was, how educated or rich she was, how well she took care of herself, how vigilant she was about having mammograms or doing breast self-examinations, or what her genetic inheritance was. Breast cancer didn't care.

She was invited to speak before the Suffolk County Legislature. Legislator Alan Binder, head of the Suffolk County Health Committee and among the few politicians who was on board early in his support of progressive legislation, had invited his mother to the hearing. She was shocked to learn about the many young women who were being diagnosed, and she praised Lorraine for making people aware of the importance of early detection. A couple of months later, when Binder was on vacation, his mother decided to have a mammogram. When he returned, she had some news for him: she had breast cancer, caught early by her mammogram.

At the same time, hundreds of women on Long Island were being diagnosed with breast cancer, but by 1994 nearly a dozen coalitions were flourishing throughout the Island. The increasing number of elected officials who were taking up the cudgels of the fight for funding and legislation made many women feel less isolated and more hopeful.

Nevertheless, in what appeared to be a cohesive effort by breast cancer advocates to politicize their agenda and to present the armor of a united front, there were increasingly obvious chinks, including the same kind of rancor and competition routinely observed in corporate America but that struck the public – who associated cancer patients with all that is high-minded and philosophically evolved – as alien and alienating.

The unity myth was revealed as early as 1992 when Geri Barish and Fran Kritchek took over the reins of 1 in 9. Housed at Adelphi, the organization felt constrained by the university. Although 1 in 9 ultimately found a temporary home at Touro Law School in Huntington, the group remained at Adelphi for over a year, agreeing to change locations only after lawyers told Barish and Kritchek that 1 in 9 had the legal right to take with them the coalition's paperwork and files, and a Tree of Life sculpture that had been presented by teachers from the Wantagh school in honor of Marie Quinn, who had worked at the school along with Kritchek.

During this time, it had become obvious to everyone that there was no love lost between Barish and the Adelphi program's director, Barbara Balaban. Each was powerful in her own right, and their clash of egos and agendas would continue for years.

Ultimately, approximately 50 women from the Adelphi support group joined 1 in 9, saying goodbye to Adelphi through clenched teeth as they were made to pay for removing the Tree of Life from the wall on which it hung.

When the Kitchen Revolutionaries came on the scene, they initially had harmonious relationships with both 1 and 9 and Adelphi, each faction supporting one another's different but also mutual efforts. It wasn't long, however, before each group found itself competing for the same things – media attention, public recognition, funding, and political allies.

In many ways, it was a horse race. Balaban didn't have breast cancer, which would have made her the least sympathetic figure if it were not for her formidable intellect, her grasp of the most complicated clinical issues, her political savvy, her affiliation with a well-regarded university, and her tireless and aggressive advocacy. When she spoke clearly about complex legislation, developed and conducted write-in campaigns, spearheaded major events, and confronted elected officials, people responded affirmatively.

Barish, an earthy, full-figured woman in her mid-40s, had flaming red hair that curled around her shoulders and a Bronx accent familiar and endearing to many transplanted Long Islanders. She told a story that made even cynics weep. Married to the love of her life at 18, she had spent her years on Long Island raising her sons, Michael and Eric. When Michael was diagnosed with Hodgkin's disease at the age of 12 and began arduous chemotherapy and radiation treatments, Geri joined the fight against cancer with a vengeance. Two weeks before Michael died at the age of 25, Geri was diagnosed with breast cancer. And not long after, on what would have been Michael's 26th birthday, her husband, Alan, suffered a debilitating stroke that relegated him permanently to a wheelchair. When she talked about cancer, about finding answers, about survival, people listened.

Lorraine represented "Everywoman" – a sympathetic figure that most people identified with when she spoke of her befuddlement at having gotten cancer and her suspicion that "something" in the environment may have caused it. When she challenged the powers-that-be by starting her own research project, the public applauded.

As an adult in college she had studied the "100th monkey" phenomenon. In the 1950s, scientists in Japan were observing monkeys on an island and dropped raw sweet potatoes in the sand for them to eat. The monkeys liked the potatoes but found the dirt unpleasant. One of the younger monkeys discovered that she could wash the dirt off, and she taught this trick to her mother and to her playmates, who in turn taught it to their mothers. For the next six years, the scientists observed that only the adults with offspring learned this innovative behavior; the other adult monkeys continued to eat the dirty potatoes.

When a certain number of monkeys had learned the washing technique – the number is actually unknown, but for purposes of explanation 100 was chosen – every monkey in the tribe almost immediately began washing their potatoes. Even more amazing is that once this critical threshold was reached, potato washing began to be observed in colonies of monkeys across the sea – monkeys who had no contact with the original monkeys!

The phenomenon was thus extrapolated to human beings: when only a limited of number of people know a new way of doing something, that knowledge remains in their purview alone. But when that number increases to a "critical mass," the new awareness may be communicated from mind to mind!

This is what appeared to happen on Long Island, where dozens and then hundreds of women were talking about breast cancer and then – in what seemed at the time to be sheer coincidence but actually may have been related to the unproven but provocative 100th monkey theory – three powerful women "discovered" breast cancer activism at almost the same time.

What Balaban, Barish, and Pace had in common was the desire to put breast cancer "on the map," unite women in powerful lobbying groups and various organizational activities, offer support, raise funds, and ultimately find a cause and cure for the disease. Balaban concentrated her energies on political action, Barish on fighting for environmental reforms and raising funds for genetic research (and in later years, founding Hewlett House, a first-of-its-kind center for cancer patients on Long Island that featured art therapy and bereavement, crisis-intervention, and support groups, et al), and Pace on mapping the "clusters" of breast cancer patients in West Islip. However, the lines were not clearly drawn, and all of them – and their followers – often found themselves fighting for the same things.

At the same time, a number of other coalitions were being established, each one unique in its own way but also similar to the original groups in the power of their leadership and their embrace of a political agenda, fund-raising efforts, and a united call for a new study.

That there is power in numbers is irrefutable, and Long Island's proliferating breast cancer movement proved the point. As increasing numbers of women rose at four in the morning to board buses for Albany and Washington, as signatures on their petitions reached into the hundreds and then thousands, and as recognized environmental groups joined their efforts, politicians took note, not with polite form letters but with aggressive and progressive legislation.

All this might have been – indeed, should have been – thrilling to the activists. But there are just so many politicians and just so much money and just so much newsprint and media minutes devoted to any one issue, and vying for these precious resources became ferocious.

The Ripple Effect

At the same time as Lorraine's project was gaining momentum, 1 in 9 instituted the Michael Scott Barish Sand Soccer tournament to raise funds for genetic research. The first contest yielded $20,000, which was donated to the Cold Spring Harbor Laboratory on Long Island in an elaborate ceremony that had flashbulbs popping.

The laboratory's illustrious leader was Dr. James D. Watson, who had won the Nobel Prize at the age of 26 – along with his colleagues Francis H. C. Crick, Maurice Wilkins (and contributor Rosalind Franklin) – for the discovery of the double helix configuration of the DNA molecule. The discovery, which promised to unlock the "secrets of life," ushered in the golden age of molecular biology and led to the Human Genome Project, an international effort under the auspices of the National Institutes of Health, to map and sequence all the genes that account for human characteristics, including disease.

Watson, widely acclaimed as "the father of genetic research," headed the Genome Project from 1988 to 1992, when the job was taken over by a former professor at Harvard Medical School. But he remained director (and then Chancellor) of Cold Spring Harbor Laboratory and was on hand to receive 1 in 9's check and to earmark the funds (which would grow to over a million dollars over the years) for a special project to study the genes that accounted for cancer.

During this time, Balaban's position as director of the Adelphi support group program and statewide hotline put her on the front line of a variety of initiatives, one of which was mobilizing support to press state legislators to pass legislation requiring that insurance companies cover screening mammograms, that medical test results be reported to patients directly, and that diagnoses and treatments for the uninsured be provided. She represented the Long Island community at the Center for Disease Control's review of study data by epidemiologists in Atlanta, helped launch the National Action Plan on Breast Cancer, and, as one of the first members of the National Breast Cancer Coalition, coordinated the organization's effort in New York State to collect 2.6 million signatures requesting more money for breast cancer research.

In truth, members of the West Islip group, 1 in 9, and Adelphi, as well as women who were forming groups of their own, were all – to greater or lesser degrees –working on these things at the same time. On the plus side, their success in making their case to politicians and scientists was empowering and helped many women speak up to their doctors and express their needs and expectations to their employers and families. They were "doing something" about breast cancer and, in a very real way, "making a difference" for future generations.

But instead of mutual praise and a spirit of solidarity, their constant struggle for money and publicity created an atmosphere of competition, mistrust, and secrecy. A "me first" mentality arose, with each group claiming to have "initiated" or "spearheaded" this or that idea or project. Often, projects that might have been more effective with the collective effort of *all* the groups resulted in each individual group essentially reinventing the wheel.

Yet the struggle to find the causes of and cure for breast cancer went on and even grew stronger. The reason, according to Barbara Balaban, could be explained by "simple arithmetic."

"Known risk factors account for 25 percent of breast cancer," she never tired of explaining, "and genetics for about 10 percent. That leaves about 65 percent unaccounted for, and women want to know why." Another number she cited proved equally chilling: every 12 minutes, breast cancer claims the life of another woman in this country. And she would note another sobering statistic: since 1960, more women have died of breast cancer than during all the wars in the history of the United States.

In spite of the brewing battles, the ripple effect continued. Donna Ketcham, who had fielded the telephone calls for the mapping project, was so deeply affected by the stories she heard that she started going to breast cancer rallies and meeting women in their 20s and 30s who had been diagnosed.

"I knew there had to be something in the environment that was causing all this cancer," she said, "because all these young women hadn't lived long enough to *do* anything to cause it."

After she married Lorraine's son in 1995, Donna suffered a miscarriage. When she read an article saying that high iron content in water could prove fatal to a developing fetus, she suspected that "the disgusting, orange water" she was drinking and bathing in might have caused her to lose the baby.

Taking a page from the Kitchen Revolutionaries, "who weren't afraid to ask questions," she consulted her doctors about the idea, but "they dismissed it out of hand."

Some ripples were disastrous. As the mapping project was drawing to an end, Maria Diorio's 32-year-old daughter-in-law, Pam Chapman Diorio, underwent a double mastectomy and had her ovaries removed. A grade school teacher, Pam had been brought up in West Islip, and she had no doubt that the toxic water from the Great South Bay was implicated in her breast cancer.

Lorraine never dreamed that when she threw the "pebble" of her idea for mapping her own community into the murky waters of Long Island, it would become the tsunami it became. In spite of that fact, by the end of 1993, the results of the survey had not yet been analyzed, and it was the analysis, Lorraine knew, that was more important than anything else.

Chapter Seven

Pieces of the Puzzle

At the same time the Kitchen Revolutionaries were marking their map on Lorraine's kitchen table, they were consulting almost constantly with Roger Grimson and asking his advice.

Dr. Grimson was an associate professor of biostatistics at the State University at Stony Brook and had spent his entire professional life analyzing scientific data and teaching his students to do the same. A 1964 graduate of the University of North Carolina at Chapel Hill, the Tar Heel State native earned a doctorate in mathematics (with an emphasis on statistics) at Duke University and completed post-doctoral work in biostatistics at UNC, where he taught the subject until he moved to Long Island and began teaching at Stony Brook in 1983.

At Stony Brook, Dr. Grimson was a colleague of Dr. Andre Varma, one of the chief investigators in the first Long Island Breast Cancer Study that was instituted in 1985 and that had concluded, just a couple of years before Lorraine's diagnosis, that the Island's high incidence of the disease was the result of the region's large Jewish population and high incomes.

Dr. Grimson had followed this and other studies that led to similar conclusions, but none of them were entirely credible to him. In the South, he had worked with a colleague whose 30-year-old wife had died from breast cancer. And on Long Island, he knew numerous women with breast cancer who didn't fit the "risk" profile even remotely. Besides, as a Long Island resident, he felt strongly that his wife was at risk and that his daughters, simply because they were female, were also at risk.

Right from the beginning, Dr. Grimson regarded the project as a complex puzzle. One piece – the major piece – was answering the mystery of West Islip's high incidence of breast cancer. But in dealing with the disparate personalities and competing priorities of the women, administrators, state officials, and members of the media, it was clear to him that there were also political, psychological, and even public relations pieces that fit into the grand scheme, and that keeping his eyes fixed on the science of the project would be his greatest challenge.

He loved the challenge! Academic science was riveting to him. But the lifelong overachiever liked people as well and was always on the lookout, he said, to find ways to "connect science to real live people." He plunged into the mapping project with high energy and keen curiosity, the same qualities that had compelled him, at age 17, to get his solo pilot's license. Although he had not pursued flying, he saw it as a metaphor for understanding the hugeness of the world and ultimately the mysteries of science.

Dr. Grimson was accustomed to juggling numerous activities – teaching, writing voluminous articles for professional journals, creating bountiful flower gardens at his Stony Brook home, and writing poetry. The youthful, good-looking 50-year-old – who people often said looked like the actor Nick Nolte – came by his motivation by virtue of a formidable gene pool: his brother Baird, a year younger, was a neuro-ophthalmologist; his brother Keith, five years younger, was an art historian; his father, a doctor (whose own father had been chief justice of the Supreme Court of North Dakota), specialized in vascular surgery; and his mother was a nutritionist.

Dr. Grimson took his science seriously, but he was nothing like the stereotype of the mad scientist, sequestered in a lab, decanting secret potions from flask to beaker. He thought of himself as a "hands-on" scientist, preferring to visit the scenes he was investigating, not just analyzing data but also "getting a feel" for the environment.

Some years before, he had conducted an epidemiological study of the cancer cases of nine fairly recent graduates of Stony Brook University. He was baffled by the unsettling common denominator in the case – all the students had lived in the Irving/O'Neill residence hall, which was being called, among other things, a "sick building" and a "cancer factory."

The study included a "control" dormitory of freshmen, environmental testing, and a large survey of the students. While some mold was found in the suspect building, it revealed no evidence of radon or other carcinogenic substances. And in analyzing the cancer cases – which ranged from stomach to thyroid to bone cancer, as well as leukemia and Hodgkin's disease – it was found that they approximated the incidence of these diseases among people in their late 20s in the general population. In the end, Dr. Grimson's study ruled out the theory that a "cluster" of cancer cases could be traced to the Stony Brook dorm.

Another "cluster" Dr. Grimson investigated resulted from an anonymous call to the state health department about a number of accidents and bone fractures among elderly patients at a Suffolk County infirmary. While the quality of caretaking and the safety of the facility were taken into consideration, Dr. Grimson's study ultimately found that the fractures occurred during months when rainfall was greatest, a statistical conclusion bolstered by "biologic plausibility."

Toward the end of the mapping project's data collection, Dr. Grimson would drive to Lorraine's home once or twice a week to pick up the questionnaires. Loading boxes that grew heavier as the weeks elapsed onto the back seat of his car and into the trunk, he'd lug them up to his Stony Brook office on a handcart, sometimes chuckling at the memory of his youthful pursuits of lifting weights, boxing, and playing football, all of which had been long abandoned and replaced by long walks. But he still found himself huffing and puffing as he lined up the boxes against the wall of his third-floor office.

The office itself was unremarkable, typical of the cubicles often occupied by tenured professors, with a wall of windows overlooking an ocean-sized parking lot, carelessly stacked piles of books and professional journals, three overflowing file cabinets, a blackboard complete with broken chalk and dusty erasers, and glaring fluorescent overhead bulbs that competed with the sunlight flooding the room in all seasons. It didn't look like an office in which history would be made. But it was – if only because it was the first legitimate "grassroots" study of its kind in the world.

Dr. Grimson's first task was to sort the data into "temporal" and "spatial" categories that established a one-year time frame for the study: the dates on which the women were diagnosed with breast cancer and the residential locations of those who reported that they had breast cancer.

Actually, this was his second task. His very first challenge was to explain to the West Islip group that their theories about clusters and environmental causes for the disease would, in essence, *never* be proven.

Laypersons, he told them, think differently than scientists do. While ordinary people might be "right" in their instinctive suspicions that X factor accounts for Y outcome, that is not the way science works. Rather, he said, science is sluggish, deliberate, cautious, skeptical. Scientists are afraid of making false claims, particularly when it comes to establishing a "relationship" between, for instance, polluted water and cancer. He told them that while feedback and input from the public was important, the burden of *proof* ultimately lay in endless scientific analysis, new studies that validated old studies – and the women's endless patience.

"I know you want this now!" he told them over and over again. "But it takes a long, long time to find answers – never-ending, it seems."

As he made his case, he was relieved that the women understood what he was saying, albeit, he detected, on solely an intellectual level. But he also appreciated their skepticism and their impatience and was eager to plunge into the analysis and, as one woman urged him, to "come up with the goods."

Poring over the first thousand surveys in October of 1993, Dr. Grimson realized that a horrible oversight had taken place: the date of diagnosis had not been included in the original questionnaire. It was a crucial piece of information that might have stopped the analysis cold if it were not for the die-hard determination of the Kitchen Revolutionaries, who, groans and frustration notwithstanding, got on their telephones and called each woman who had filled out a survey. This process would delay Dr. Grimson's analysis for months.

And just as the women had been dealing constantly with unexpected glitches in their project, Dr. Grimson had a few obstacles of his own to hurdle. One day, while reading a professional journal, he came upon a Request for Proposal (RFP) notice that offered scientists an opportunity to tell the academic and science communities what kinds of research they thought was most urgently needed by society. If the proposal involved a health issue (such as cancer) and was deemed worthy of research, a request for a research grant would be sent to the National Cancer Institute for approval.

Without hesitating, Dr. Grimson and some of his Stony Brook colleagues submitted a response to the RFP informing the powers-that-be that they were working on not one but three Long Island mapping projects – West Islip, Huntington, and Babylon – and that a need for further study was urgent. Although the process of submitting a proposal and then waiting for its acceptance can be long and frustrating, Dr. Grimson was amazed and delighted to learn within months that the proposal had been accepted by the NCI – Stony Brook had gotten the grant!

If, however, everything in life is timing, as some people claim, the timing for the much-coveted grant could not have been worse since it coincided with the NCI's evolving interest in studying a possible relationship between breast cancer and the environment on Long Island. As it happened, at just about the same time that Dr. Grimson submitted his proposal, Columbia University submitted an RFP of its own, and the grant Columbia was awarded – to Dr. Grimson's consternation and fury – became the basis for the Long Island Breast Cancer Study Project (LIBCSP) for which the advocacy groups and Senator D'Amato had lobbied so vigorously.

In other words, Columbia had been selected by the NCI to be the lead investigator in the study project that would evaluate the current and past exposure of people in Nassau and Suffolk counties on Long Island (and in Schoharie County, New York, and Tolland County, Connecticut) to contaminated drinking water, sources of indoor and ambient air pollution (including aircraft emissions), pesticides and other toxic chemicals, hazardous and municipal waste, and other factors the NCI deemed appropriate.

In short order, Dr. Grimson was told that the grant he'd been awarded to investigate environmental causes of breast cancer on

Long Island was in direct conflict with the non-negotiable desires of the NCI to have Columbia perform this part of the LIBCSP.

Deflated but undaunted, he submitted another proposal to the NCI requesting that Stony Brook be in charge of investigating the possible relationship between electromagnetic fields (EMFs) and breast cancer. Numerous studies had already appeared in professional journals suggesting that higher cancer rates existed in neighborhoods with transformer boxes and power lines that emit EMFs, and a number of Long Island activists were beginning to question how the emissions related to the increasing incidence of cancer, including leukemia. Although EMFs had not been included in the NCI's original study design, Dr. Grimson convinced the organization that the study should include them and succeeded in getting Stony Brook accepted as a participant in the landmark study.

All this took time – painful, sluggish, frustrating time – which further delayed the analysis of the West Islip mapping project. By the time the data collection process for the West Islip project was complete, 5,485 questionnaires had been submitted. The data were entered onto a disk by Loop Data, Inc., of Holbrook (Long Island) and returned to Dr. Grimson so he could check for quality control and finally begin his analysis. Immediately, however, he found that a number of people had responded twice, requiring him to remove 219 records from the database, which left 5,266 analyzable records.

Time marched on. And on.

Yet there was little time to complain. Lorraine had plunged into her new job at Stony Brook and was busy setting up her new grassroots organization, Breast Cancer Help, Inc. The original West Islip group was engaging in public speaking, political forums, and fund-raising. In addition, the momentum of the breast cancer movement on Long Island was picking up speed, with new coalitions placing pressure on state health officials for new initiatives and on elected officials for increased research funding and new legislation.

They knew that lobbying Senator D'Amato was equivalent to "preaching to the choir." He had already secured $260 million – or a 165 percent increase – in federal breast cancer research funding in fiscal year 1993, and he had submitted budget estimates of $1.8 million for 1994 and $4 million for 1995. In keeping up his drumbeat of advocacy, he also had requested a six-month status report from the NCI.

The activists also knew that their presence at untold numbers of political events was mandatory, the better to reinforce their role in this or that accomplishment as well as to show support for this or that sponsor. One event took place in April of 1994 when Dr. Mark Chassin, New York state's commissioner of health, announced findings of a study that had been suggested by one of the breast cancer movement's best friends, Dr. James Melius, the director of the state's division of occupational health and environmental epidemiology.

At the urging of breast cancer patients throughout Long Island with whom he met regularly in small groups, Dr. Melius developed a study to examine the relationship of cancer to emissions of exhaust and fuel fumes at airports and major roadways. Using geographic information software, researchers divided Long Island into 5,809 "grid cells," each with an area of approximately 5.8 miles.

By drawing on data from the state's Industrial Directory, two groups of factories were identified: 75 chemical industrial plants, a group believed to be "more likely" to emit toxic air pollutants; and 650 manufacturing plants, a group considered "likely" to emit toxic air pollutants.

Dr. Chassin announced the frightening results that 14.5 percent of women living near large chemical manufacturing facilities ran the risk of developing breast cancer after menopause, but for women who did not live near such plants, the risk was only 9.5 percent. Breaking the study down further, it was found that women living near chemical plants in Nassau County ran a 62 percent higher than average risk of getting breast cancer, and in Suffolk County the risk was 61 percent – risks almost equal to having a family history of the disease.

It was an unprecedented study, one that might never have taken place were it not for the insistence of women who wanted to explore every possible reason for the escalating incidence of breast cancer in the region. Immediate follow-up to the study was begun. One of the responses was a concerted effort to require the Department of Environmental Conservation to change the regulations of the federal Clean Air Act, in essence requiring the Environmental Protection Agency to curtail the release of toxic chemicals from industries and to impose economic sanctions on firms failing to comply.

The study was a major step forward in terms of establishing a relationship between the environment and breast cancer. Just as important, it led Senator D'Amato and Republican Congressman Peter T. King to fault the NCI for denying Long Island breast cancer groups a policy-shaping role in the new Long Island Breast Cancer Study Project. The initial study of 1985 was noteworthy not only for its questionable conclusions – which ran the gamut from controversial to wrong – but also for excluding community input.

In a letter to Samuel Broder, the NCI's director, Senator D'Amato wrote, "Long Island breast cancer survivors and their families and friends were the crucial catalysts in getting the federal government to recognize the possible link between the environment and breast cancer on Long Island. Now that we are finally moving forward with this landmark study, it is outrageous that those most affected and knowledgeable are left out of the process."

It was not only the senator who was pushing for community input. From the time the NCI announced its landmark study, a number of community activists had been writing and speaking to the higher-ups at the prestigious institute, in essence warning them that a lack of communication would not be tolerated and that they would use their contacts in the press and the political world to keep insisting that regular press conferences about the progress of the study would be held and that the opinions and advice of members of the community would be factored into the process.

After a few months, there was no doubt that the NCI was listening. Dr. Iris Obrams, the director of the Long Island Breast Cancer Study Project, called the acting health commissioner of Nassau County, Dr. Abby Greenberg, asking to speak with a representative of the Breast Cancer Detection and Education Department, which was funded by a grant from the state.

She was put in touch with Ellyn Troisi, a health educator in the department who oversaw the mobile mammography van that routinely visited neighborhoods and business sites to provide women with the free screenings the county executive had mandated in the mid-1980s. Dr. Obrams explained to her that the people who were conducting the study were looking for access to the community and its leaders, the better to share information and gain input.

Ellyn responded to Dr. Obram's request with tireless enthusiasm, meeting with community groups, coalitions, governmental agencies and individuals throughout Long Island. In May of 1994, six months after the study was announced, The Long Island Breast Cancer Network was established and Ellyn was elected coordinator of the group, a position she held for two years.

But even before that, the NCI showed that it was working with the community in good faith when Karen Miller, the founder of the Huntington Breast Cancer Coalition, was chosen to be a community representative for the study project.

The competitive reaction of some of the activists to Karen's selection didn't escape Ellyn's attention, however. She knew that many of the coalitions had different political agendas and that it was her job to keep the Network members focused on the group's strictly apolitical agenda.

Network meetings began to take place every three or four months in the conference rooms of various hotels on Long Island, with NCI representatives, including principal investigator Dr. Marilee Gammon of Columbia University, always in attendance. The group's purpose was solely to exchange information about coalition activities and the study's progress, not to address political issues or raise funds.

But some attendees were leery. They suspected that the real purpose of the network was to enable representatives from the NCI to keep tabs on the work of the coalitions, in essence to make sure that the "kitchen science" the activists were engaging in didn't conflict with or gain more publicity than the institution's study.

At the first couple of Network meetings, stone-faced activists sat eyeing one another skeptically, hesitant to "share" information about the goings-on in their respective coalitions and distrustful of American Cancer Society and NCI representatives, whose role was still unclear.

Notwithstanding occasional conflicts, however, the result of the Network meetings was an unusually positive relationship between the NCI and community shakers-and-movers, who came to believe they finally had direct access to a large and often historically inaccessible governmental agency.

Just as important, many of the internecine battles and fierce competition that had characterized the coalitions were ameliorated when members of the Network realized, according to Ellyn Troisi, that "there was more strength in numbers and that we all had the same goal – getting closer to the causes of breast cancer."

"Getting closer," to each member of the Network and to other activists on Long Island, meant getting answers. But the NCI study had just begun and no one expected that it would yield any answers for years to come. No one was more aware of this than Dr. Grimson, who was working feverishly to complete his first analysis of the West Islip survey.

A month after the Network was founded – in June of 1994 – the Kitchen Revolutionaries collected their last survey and sent it to Dr. Grimson. It had been almost two years since the mapping project was begun. In that time, the lives of the West Islip participants had been transformed, not only by their illnesses but also by their activism and by life itself. Now busy as ever with the political and community activities of the WIBCC, they heaved a collective sigh of relief, anticipating that Dr. Grimson's analysis would confirm their suspicions and redeem their efforts.

The West Islip women had total faith in Roger Grimson and had worked with him harmoniously since the beginning of the mapping project. But as the months dragged on, some of them began to wonder if "politics as usual" – specifically, pressure from the NCI to *not* "come up with the answers" – had something to do with the impossible amount of time it was taking him to complete his analysis.

That was not the case at all, Dr. Grimson told them, explaining that analyzing scientific data was a time-consuming process and that the NCI study would probably take a lot longer than its projected five years (which it did) and also that their analysis might take even longer!

It was hard for Lorraine and the other women not to believe the earnest scientist, who one Kitchen Revolutionary benevolently labeled "the absent-minded professor." They appreciated the pressure he was under, including the fact that publicity about the mapping project had gained international notoriety and that, using the West Islip project as a model, people in England, Poland, and Hiroshima, Japan, were mapping areas in their own countries.

To deal with their frustration, many of the women began to resort to pregnancy jokes. "Isn't this baby awfully overdue?' one woman asked, while another said, "Let's give Roger a little castor oil and induce this baby!"

Finally, on March 8, 1995 (significantly, nine months after he received the last survey), Dr. Grimson delivered "the baby" – his long-awaited analysis.

To the excitement of the West Islip group and, in fact, all Long Islanders, the report was published and released to the public. A portion of the study confirmed what they already knew: that known breast cancer risks such as family history and age were, in fact, related to the occurrence of the disease. Two interesting findings were that women who had used birth control pills had a lower rate of breast cancer than those who had not, and that women who had breast-fed their children had less breast cancer than those who had not.

But all this was moot to the women who knew that the whole point of the study was to determine if there were clusters of breast cancer in West Islip. To that end, Linda Timander, a master's degree student in the geography department of Hunter College in New York City, who was writing her thesis on the mapping project under the partial guidance of Dr. Grimson, had constructed maps of long-term residents in West Islip, which included women with and without breast cancer.

In addition, the Babylon, Long Island, firm of Greenman-Pederson was hired to create a geographic information system (GIS) upon which the maps of the area were based. A GIS can store, manipulate, and analyze data as well as display the relationships between geographic locations. It can look for factors associated with public health issues and be used to map potential sources of pollution, both past and present, that researchers can study for a possible association with breast cancer patterns. Some have compared the system to an updated version of the old World Book Encyclopedia maps that had Mylar sheets overlying one another, each one revealing a different facet of a particular area, for instance political divisions, crops and vegetation, population density, the list goes on.

Some of the overlays in the mapping project that Dr. Grimson was analyzing involved geographic and health information as well as the all-important variables of environment, the locations of factories and other potential sources of pollution, and clusters.

The release of the study, however, disappointed the West Islip group, which thought Dr. Grimson's analysis was "interesting" but too full of terms such as multivariate analysis and nonparametric methods and p-values and not full enough of the "proof" they wanted that clusters existed. It was little consolation to the women that his second and final analysis would not be forthcoming for several months.

Dr. Grimson remembered the WIBCC member who had urged him to "come up with some answers," and he sensed that both the public and the NCI were looking in his direction. Not just looking, but also, in the case of the Kitchen Revolutionaries, calling him frequently to find out his "timetable." Dr. Grimson was preoccupied with his teaching and consulting duties, however, and with increasing participation in the mapping projects of other communities and with getting Stony Brook's EMF study off the ground. The best he could do was promise the women that he was putting his "best efforts" into completing the second analysis.

If any doubts about Dr. Grimson's timetable remained, they were finally dispelled when the completion of the second analysis was announced at a large press conference at Good Samaritan Hospital in November of 1995 – eight months after the first analysis and nearly three and a half years after the survey first appeared on the front page of *Suffolk Life*.

From its opening paragraph, the report that Dr. Grimson distributed in booklet form – to *Newsday* reporters (including Dan Fagin who had written extensively about breast cancer on Long Island in a number of award-winning articles), N.J. Burkett of Channel 7 Eyewitness News, a swarm of other media, state officials, medical people, and West Islip Breast Cancer Coalition members – made clear that the estimated age-adjusted breast cancer incidence in West Islip for the years 1978–1987 (the last available data from New York state) was 86 per 1,000, which was *lower* than most other community rates in Suffolk and Nassau counties.

The women didn't quite know how to interpret this finding, but they reasoned that even if the study showed no clusters, they still would have succeeded in bringing the possible breast cancer-environment connection to the public – the proof being that the NCI was now on Long Island looking at that very possibility!

Dr. Grimson's report confirmed this notion by stating unequivocally that the rationale for the mapping project was to yield useful epidemiological and geographic information about the disease. "If initiators or promoters of breast cancer are associated (at least for many cases) with residential location," he said, "then the maps included in the analysis may suggest hypotheses about key environmental factors."

The only eligibility requirement for the survey was that every woman who responded had to be a resident of West Islip and at least 25 years old. GIS was used to create 12 maps displaying such data as the length of time a woman had lived at her residence – for instance, one or more years, 10 or more years, 15 or more years, 20 or more years, 25 or more years, and 30 or more years. A home in which breast cancer had been diagnosed was colored blue, and a home in which no diagnosis had been made was colored yellow. The locations of those who didn't respond were left uncolored.

The maps provided the women who answered the survey with a guarantee of as much confidentiality as possible considering that the locations of their homes would be color-coded on the map of West Islip and ostensibly available to anyone curious enough to do some investigating. And they provided Dr. Grimson with, among other things, a history of residency for long-term and non-cases of breast cancer (which is helpful in pattern or cluster analysis) and also an ability to deduce landmarks such as industrial plants and other potential sources of pollution.

In many cases, the surveys failed to determine the dates of diagnoses, which Dr. Grimson considered problematic. But he decided that omitting this information would "not introduce bias that would falsely show a different geographic pattern between cases and non-cases" and that learning the total length of residency was adequate to go forward with his analysis. In addition, several men whose homes were not included in the analysis responded to the survey, revealing that their wives had died of breast cancer.

The West Islip group was particularly concerned with data about the area south of Montauk Highway, where all of them lived. They rushed through the first six pages of the report until they reached "RESULTS," which included a review of the study's hypotheses and conclusions.

The first hypothesis was that breast cancer was more apt to occur among women who lived on or near dead-end streets than among those who lived elsewhere. Dead-end streets were a concern because most of them had dead-end water mains in which the flow of water was delayed and therefore more susceptible to contamination.

> The report verified that breast cancer risk was higher among women who lived on or near dead-end streets *south* of Montauk Highway.

The second hypothesis was that breast cancer occurred more frequently among long-term residents who lived near the Dzus Fastener Company, a manufacturing plant in operation between 1932 and 1985. The plant produced electroplating and metal cleaning wastes that were discharged into a series of dry wells and a leach field, effectively releasing cadmium, chromium, and cyanide into the soil and groundwater.

The report did not confirm this hypothesis, noting that the company was located on the north side of Union Boulevard and west of the vertical center of West Islip.

The third hypothesis was that breast cancer was more prevalent among women living south of Montauk Highway than among women residing north of Montauk Highway. The east-west highway divides West Islip into a northerly region and a smaller southerly region near the Great South Bay.

The report confirmed this hypothesis, noting that among all long-term respondents, a greater proportion (4.2 percent) of women with a history of breast cancer lived *south* of Montauk Highway than north of the highway (3.2 percent). For those who had lived for at least 20 years at their current addresses, the proportions north and south of the highway were 5.0 percent and 8.4 percent, respectively. For those who had lived at least 30 years at their current addresses, the proportions were 5.7 percent and 11.3 percent.

The report stated that women living south of the highway were "more affluent on average" than those north of it, affluence being a known "risk factor" for breast cancer. Strangely, however, questions of personal income or wealth were *not* included on the questionnaire that was mailed to West Islip residents.

"If the analysis removes [certain] factors and other potential confounders or potential biases," the report stated, "then the geographic difference must be attributed to either local geographically based environmental factors or to a broader spectrum of environmental matters that may involve diet and/or other social or life-style factors that differ between long-term residents living north and south of Montauk Highway."

Doctors, scientists, and lay people all over Long Island were keenly interested in Dr. Grimson's report, many of them having suspected that clusters of breast cancer existed in numerous communities and not just in West Islip. To them, there was now "proof." But even though great numbers of them believed that the clusters pointed to the fact that "something" in the environment was causing so much cancer, they were still hard put to say what it was.

Dr. Grimson was aware that the survey was the first-ever small-area breast cancer study and that both the lay public and seasoned researchers were intensely curious about its findings. But analytical scientist that he was, and is, he spelled out in his analysis the impossibility of identifying any particular environmental causes in such a limited, population-based study.

"It is important to realize that the survey questionnaire was *not* designed to *determine* environmental causes of breast cancer," he stated on the report's second page, explaining that "the enormous objectives of determining new factors associated with breast cancer requires extensive questionnaires, home visits by a team of experts, measurements of amounts of hypothesized exposures, blood and urine samples, and much more," which would cost "millions of dollars."

In contrast, his study – for which Stony Brook received $20,000 – involved a one-page questionnaire, no home visits by teams of experts, no environmental or human sampling, and, by any measure, the shortest of shoestring budgets.

However, the limitations of the study – including the fact that many respondents hadn't recorded the date when their breast cancer was diagnosed – were far outweighed by the illuminating results that it yielded.

In addition to gaining international recognition, the Kitchen Revolutionaries had inspired numerous local and national grassroots groups to begin their own mapping projects, and they had been key players in inspiring the NCI to commit to "the enormous objectives of determining new (specifically environmental) factors associated with breast cancer" by coming to Long Island and establishing the multi-year, multimillion-dollar Long Island Breast Cancer Study Project.

Of the 8,740 surveys that were distributed to the West Islip community, 5,082 were returned, a noteworthy, statistically significant 65 percent that gave the results scientific credibility and which Dr. Grimson described as "excellent."

Astonishingly, the survey picked up 400 women with malignancies and 800 with benign tumors, many of whom had been either inspired or frightened into going for mammographies when the questionnaire was published and they realized that their own community might be a "hot spot."

The West Islip group was exultant. While the release of the analysis brought the mapping project to an end, all of them felt that the more than 2,000 hours they had spent collecting and collating survey data had raised public awareness about clusters, breast cancer, and the environment beyond their wildest dreams.

"We're doing it with tobacco," exclaimed Ginny Regnante when she read the analysis, referring to the fight by health activists to get the powers-that-be to concede that tobacco was deadly, "and we're doing it with breast cancer and the environment!"

Equally, if not more, beside herself was Lorraine. In announcing the results of the analysis, Dr. Grimson publicly cited Lorraine, describing as "astute" the original observations she had made more than three years earlier. She was gratified by the acknowledgment but also overwhelmed by the realization that her brainchild had officially come to an end. While she and the other women would continue, relentlessly, to carry on their battle for answers, at that moment she felt like fleeing the reporters, the cameras, the general hoopla, and her own celebrity, and running off to be by herself.

When she got home at 5:30, she noted 22 messages on her answering machine. Ignoring them, she stepped out of her heels,

222

steeped herself a cup of chamomile tea, and put on a bulky woolen sweater. She carried the hot brew – and Dr. Grimson's analysis – to the expansive wooden porch off her kitchen. It was an atypically balmy night for November, and the water of the Great South Bay that lay before her seemed unusually still and peaceful.

Lorraine intended to read every word of the analysis that evening and to contemplate its full meaning. Instead, she found herself gazing at the darkening skyline and thinking back to the long, hard road that had brought her to this point: learning of her terrifying diagnosis, walking around her neighborhood and meeting 20 other women with breast cancer, suspecting that she was living in a cluster of breast cancer, and then resolving to find out if her suspicions were accurate.

She remembered her exhilaration at learning that Lou Grasso would publish the survey on the front page of *Suffolk Life*'s West Islip issue, the anxiety she and the other Kitchen Revolutionaries experienced when a shortage of money made it look as if the project would go nowhere, the arduous but successful lobbying trips to Washington and Albany, the blur of speaking engagements and interviews, and the tremendous intelligence and passion the women across Long Island had brought to the fight against breast cancer. And she remembered the many women – both close friends and strangers – who had lost their lives to the disease or were still battling to stay alive.

Lorraine shuddered as the darkness enveloped her and the air turned chilly. As she rose to go back into the house, she noticed that the sky was filled with twinkling stars. Mesmerized by the sight, she focused on one that was particularly bright, addressing the star as she had so many audiences.

"As long as you're shining, as long as there's one ray of light, one hope to find the answer to breast cancer," she intoned to the darkness, "I'll keep on going."

Then she entered her house to listen to her phone messages.

Afterword

In the years since 1994, when Lorraine Pace and her neighbors completed mapping the hamlet of West Islip, breast cancer activism on Long Island has continued unabated. Many of the early participants – and leaders – in the grassroots coalitions who are mentioned in this book remain at the forefront, having successfully lobbied for:

- An updated New York state tumor registry and the expansion of the state's Breast Cancer Registry.
- A statewide pesticide registry.
- The passage of the New York state Neighborhood Notification law, which requires 48-hour notice to notify neighbors before the spraying of any pesticide.
- The passage of the New York state Pesticide Registry law, which bans the use of pesticides on new golf courses.
- A family breast and ovarian cancer registry.
- The posting of maps of cancer rates in every ZIP code in New York state on the Department of Health's website.
- The passage of a law that ends "drive-through" mastectomies to insure that only a woman and her doctor determine when discharge from the hospital after breast surgery is indicated, and mandates that insurance companies provide coverage for reconstructive surgery.
- The passage of a law requiring clinical breast exams by a physician when a mammography is performed.
- Various initiatives focusing on increased research funding, public education, and better breast cancer treatment.

Over the years, Lorraine testified personally before numerous congressional, state and local hearings regarding the possible link between breast cancer and the environment. In addition, the group she founded, Breast Cancer Help, Inc., opened the Long Island Cancer Help and Wellness Center in Lindenhurst, with Lynda Distler (a former mayor of Lindenhurst) as the Executive Director. The center offers programs to increase awareness and promote early detection, as well as providing cancer patients with psychosocial support and programs such as yoga, art therapy and massage therapy.

Lorraine introduced the director of The Long Island Cancer Center at Stony Brook, Dr. Jack Kovach, to Babylon Town Supervisor, Steve Bellone, in order to establish The Witness Project in Babylon, which provides early detection and support to African-American women who have breast cancer.

Breast Cancer Help also raised over a million and a half dollars to obtain the most cutting-edge medical equipment in the region. With the help of Suffolk County Executive Robert Gaffney and county legislator Cameron Alden, Breast Cancer Help purchased the first two of three modules for the Novalis radio-surgery system for Stony Brook University Medical Center, where the organization also helped establish a toll-free cancer HELPLINE.

The organization was at the forefront of the passage of several important laws. One of them, introduced by State Senator Kemp Hannon, with assistance from Dr. Roger Grimson and Kathy Porchia, a Cancer Registry registrar, mandated that only certified registrars enter cancer data into hospital registries. Another law, introduced by New York State Assemblyman Robert Sweeney, allows breast cancer patients to adopt children. Yet another, introduced by State Senator Kenneth LaValle and supported by activist Joan Therese Hudson and the Suffolk County Breast Health Partnership, addresses education about breast cancer and testicular cancer. And the " Give a Gift to Breast Cancer" check-off on the New York State Income Tax Form enables taxpayers to contribute to the New York State Breast Cancer Research and Education Fund.

Continuing its collaboration with Stony Brook University Medical Center, Breast Cancer Help helped to obtain, through the efforts of former U.S. Congressman Michael Forbes, $5 million for the Long Island Cancer Center at Stony Brook. And with the assistance of former U.S. Congressman Felix Grucci, Breast Cancer Help worked to procure $1 million for the Long Island Cancer Database Project at Stony Brook.

In addition, Breast Cancer Help spearheaded a $500,000, 63-month lease for the GE Digital Mammography system at Stony Brook University Hospital, which was facilitated by a $250,000 grant from State Senator Caesar Trunzo to help with the payments of $7,000 per month.

Breast Cancer Help also donated half the funds for the Confirma CADStream MRI Reader that is used at the Long Island Cancer Center at Stony Brook University Hospital to assist radiologists in providing improved diagnoses of breast cancer.

And along with the New York State Grand Lodge Order Sons of Italy, Breast Cancer Help donated funds to Cold Spring Harbor Laboratory for the purchase of a confocal laser scanning microscope that allows researchers to view breast cancer cells three dimensionally.

In 1994, Lorraine and Breast Cancer Help worked with Alex Fezza (a member of the organization's board of directors) to spearhead a major letter-writing campaign that succeeded in changing federal regulations to provide insurance coverage for stem-cell infusion therapy for federal employees. And in the mid-1990s the advocacy group also helped to obtain $80,000 from State Assemblyman Paul Harenburg to improve prostate cancer and breast cancer care in the Department of Radiation and Oncology at Stony Brook University Hospital.

And to make it easy for businesses and local residents to join in the fight against breast cancer, the organization instituted the Breast Cancer Help Clothing Bin campaign, with over 200 drop locations throughout Long Island.

In addition, Lorraine met dozens of amazing women who faced the challenge of breast cancer in unique and inspiring ways. Among them was Maureen McGrory DiPalma – an active member of the Breast Cancer Help board until she died of the disease in 2000 – who worked tirelessly to raise funds for the diagnostic and treatment equipment at Stony Brook Hospital and – through her position at Grand Union Supermarkets and with the backing of Teen Life, a Catholic youth group – to establish a walk in her community of Lindenhurst.

Now well into the 21ˢᵗ century, the original board members of Breast Cancer Help are still active, and the organization has a number of new members who have expanded and diversified its role, for instance oncology nurse Lillian Morales, who represents the Hispanic community, and Doris Weisman, a nurse practitioner and women's health advocate. And Lorraine herself continues her tradition of activism, among other activities representing Breast Cancer Help, Inc. on Suffolk County Executive Steve Levy's Cancer Task Force.

"But none of the all-important legislative accomplishments of Breast Cancer Help or the other grassroots coalitions would ever have been realized," Lorraine says, "if it hadn't been for the ongoing support and advocacy of New York's Governor, George Pataki, and his willingness to sign the legislation and throw the full force of his influence behind it."

Lorraine said she felt "blessed" with four granddaughters. "After I was diagnosed, I never dreamed I'd ever live long enough to have them in my life." She has also been responsible for starting over 25 coalitions in the United States. In a 1996 special cancer edition of *Scientific American*, she was the first-ever layperson to be featured in the prestigious magazine, and she participated in an HBO special, "Rachel's Daughters," produced by Allie and Irving Light, and in "Say It, Fight It, Cure It," produced by Lee Grant for Lifetime Television.

However, the study of the possible relationship between breast cancer and the environment that Lorraine, her colleagues, and other activists relentlessly lobbied for during the early 1990s turned out to yield significantly less information than they had anticipated.

When Congress passed a law in March 1993 mandating that the National Cancer Institute undertake the massive Long Island Breast Cancer Study Project – which was originally earmarked at $10 million over a period of five years – the entire country seemed hopeful that at least a few rays of light would be shed on the environment's role in escalating cancer rates in every corner of the United States.

The law that Senator Al D'Amato had made the cornerstone – indeed, the mission – of his service to his constituents was actually written by Phil Schiliro, a longtime aide to liberal Rep. Henry Waxman of California (the chair of the House subcommittee on health and the environment). The law specified which subjects would be studied and who would conduct the research.

But instead of the project being placed under the jurisdiction of the government's chief research institution, the National Institutes of Health, Congress granted the project to one of NIH's subsidiaries, the National Cancer Institute, over which Waxman's committee had direct budget authority. This decision effectively excluded institutions more closely associated with environmental issues, such as the Environmental Protection Agency and the National Institute of Environmental Health Sciences.

The NCI's mandate was crystal clear: (1) to conduct a case-control study in which approximately 3,000 women with breast cancer would be compared with a control group of cancer-free women; (2) to study environmental factors that might contribute to the incidence of breast cancer, looking specifically at contaminated drinking water, electromagnetic fields, pesticides and hazardous waste, air pollution, and "other factors" to be selected by the science institute; and (3) to develop a GIS (geographic information system) to map possible links between cancer cases and polluted sites.

The NCI researchers, under the supervision of Dr. G. Iris Obrams, spent a year planning the 12 studies that the study project would include, but even then she questioned the design of the study. She believed that the case-control model that studies sick people and compares them to well people would be less effective than a longitudinal study that tracked a large group of people for years – breast cancer can develop over 20 years – looking at genes, environmental factors, and patterns of behavior that might explain the origins of the disease process.

In 1994, Dr. Marilee Gammon was selected to head the Long Island study. An associate professor of epidemiology at Columbia University, she had already conducted large case-control studies in New Jersey and New York City. The following year, in January of 1995, she received approval for the major part of the Long Island Breast Cancer Study Project: an $8 million study comparing the environmental exposures of women with breast cancer and cancer-free women.

Throughout the planning process, however, Senator D'Amato complained to the NCI that local activists on Long Island – the people who had spearheaded the study – were being left out of the loop. Finally, in March of 1995, the NCI named four lay activists to its 13-member scientific advisory board.

But Senator D'Amato and his constituents were still not satisfied and accused the NCI of earmarking a whopping 25 percent of the study's funds for research on nutrition, family history of breast cancer, and ways to encourage more women to get mammograms, all of which, he said, were unrelated to the environment.

It seemed that every step of the way was fraught with grievances and arguments. When Dr. Gammon decided to limit the chemicals to be tested in the blood and urine of her study's subjects to already-banned products such as DDT, dieldrin, chlordane, and PCBs, the Long Island activists were furious, having expected that there would be more concentration on household products and pesticides. Dr. Gammon's study did look at the byproducts of such items as cigarettes and fuel.

For years, the unwieldy project dragged on, with both laypersons and scientists questioning the appropriateness of the geographic information system, personnel being ousted or replaced, and the public growing weary and also wary about the outcome.

At the beginning of 1996, Dr. Gammon began to interview the subjects of her study. By the end of the year, the cost of the LIBCSP had ballooned to an estimated $30 million. It took another year for Dr. Gammon to finish collecting her data and yet two more to complete her laboratory work. And it wasn't until 1999 that the NCI hired Virginia-based AverStar Inc. to begin building a GIS database for the study project – six years after Congress ordered the system.

By 2001, no results had been released to the public, and it didn't help matters that articles Gammon submitted to *The Journal of the American Medical Association* and the *Journal of the National Cancer Institute* had been rejected because peer reviewers had issued negative commentaries about her study and a number of scientists already were contradicting her conclusions.

In August of 2002 – almost a decade after Congress mandated the project – Gammon's study was finally released to the public in an article published in the journal *Cancer Epidemiology, Biomarkers & Prevention*. Its conclusion – *no evidence that pollution in general or the four banned chemicals that were tested specifically caused breast cancer in Long Island women* – was shocking to the many women on Long Island who felt certain that "something" in the environment was causing so many of them to get breast cancer.

The study also found that breast cancer was 50 percent more likely in women who were exposed to a group of compounds found in cigarette smoke, fuel exhaust, and charbroiled foods, but that statistic left many scientists unconvinced.

Another startling finding was that, contrary to popular thinking on Long Island, the region's breast cancer rate was *lower* than the national average, including such places as San Francisco, Seattle, and Atlanta.

All in all, the study project was disappointing to the activists, but not discouraging in terms of their ongoing battle to fulfill their oft-stated mission to find "a cause and a cure" for the dreaded disease.

While they expressed frustration, even anger, with the length of time the study had taken and, as one activist opined, "all of its non-conclusions," most viewed the very existence of the study in a positive light, not only citing the advances in biology, genetics, and computing that had occurred over the previous decade but also, and especially, feeling pride in the special role they had played in capturing the attention of the powers-that-be in the world of politics and scientific research and placing the still-mysterious link between breast cancer and the environment on the front burner of public consciousness.

"We didn't expect miracles, and we didn't get the magic bullet we hoped for," Lorraine said about the study's conclusions. "But breast cancer had taught all of us that progress is only won with a fight. And our fight is far from over."

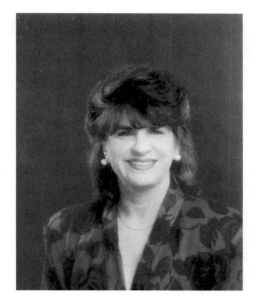

JOAN SWIRSKY, a longtime writer for The New York Times and numerous other publications, is the recipient of seven Long Island Press awards. A former obstetrical nurse and Lamaze teacher and a practicing psychotherapist, she is the author and coauthor of 10 books, including "The Breast Cancer Handbook" and "Coping with Lymphedema." She lives on Long Island with her businessman husband Steve and they have three children and three grandchildren.